"The book *The Astonishing Adolescent Upheaval in Psychoanalysis* is of great interest to any clinical psychoanalyst confronted with the issue of adolescence in the 21st century. Through different perspectives, renowned psychoanalysts of contemporary adolescence present the psychoanalytic tools they use when facing clinical situations that go beyond the emotional turmoil that is expected for this period of life."

Sergio Lewkowicz, *professor and supervisor for psychoanalytic psychotherapy in the Psychiatry Department of the Medical School of the Federal University of Rio Grande do Sul, is a psychiatrist and training and supervising psychoanalyst of the Porto Alegre Psychoanalytic Society (SPPA). He is a member of the gender and sexual diversity studies committee of the IPA.*

"This book is brilliant, exciting, and very accessible; this is a rare combination of articles and discussions from well-known psychoanalysts from all over the world, Argentina, Brazil, Canada, Italy, Switzerland, Turkey, and Uruguay. They share their complex views on adolescence, dealing in depth with psychoanalytic theory. Very interesting developments on the clinical association of isolation, violence, addiction are presented in this volume, showing the dynamics and the suffering at play from very early in life, and the economics of the drives in narcissistic organizations. Many analytic cures are presented, a rich material for thinking and education."

Christine Anzieu-Premmereur, *MD, PhD, is Assistant Clinical Professor, Psychiatry, at Columbia University, and Faculty, Columbia Psychoanalytic Center. She is also Chair of the IPA COCAP and Co-Founder of Pulsion.of Pulsion.*

W0113748

The Astonishing Adolescent Upheaval in Psychoanalysis

This book brings together international contributors to share insight from their theoretical and clinical work with adolescents, considering the different psychopathological responses they see in adolescent patients and how these can be worked with in analysis.

Each chapter addresses a specific topic, focusing on representing the clinical realities facing psychoanalysts in treating adolescents with different types of disturbances at the psychic level. They cover a range of situations and perspectives, including discussion of maternal violence, the erotic field, self-mutilation, and social withdrawal, with a core focus on issues affecting contemporary adolescents. Bringing together a vast range of experience, *The Astonishing Adolescent Upheaval in Psychoanalysis* presents a new approach which re-establishes the impact of the responses of significant objects in the impasses present in narcissistic suffering. This book will be of great interest to all psychoanalytic and psychodynamic clinicians working with adolescents.

Roosevelt Cassorla, MD, PhD, is a training analyst at the Brazilian Psychoanalytic Societies of São Paulo and Campinas. He is Full Professor at the State University of Campinas and a member of the College of The International Journal of Psychoanalysis. His recent books include *Advances in Contemporary Psychoanalytic Field Theory* (co-editor) and *The Psychoanalyst, the Theatre of Dreams and the Clinic of Enactment* (both Routledge), and *Suicide Studies: Psychoanalysis and Mental Health* (in Portuguese). He received the 2017 Mary S. Sigourney Award for Outstanding Achievement in Psychoanalysis.

Silvia Flechner, MD, is a child, adolescent, and adult training analyst at the Uruguayan Psychoanalytic Society. She is the IPA Publications Committee Chair for the term 2021–2025, and she has been a member of the Board of the International Journal of Psychoanalysis since 2008.

Psychoanalytic Ideas and Applications Series

Series Editor: Silvia Flechner

The Infinite Infantile and the Psychoanalytic Task
Psychoanalysis with Children, Adolescents and their Families
Edited by Nilde Parada Franch, Christine Anzieu-Premmereur, Mónica Cardenal and Majlis Winberg Salomonsson

A Psychoanalytic Understanding of Trauma
Post-Traumatic Mental Functioning, the Zero Process, and the Construction of Reality
Joseph Fernando

The Poetry of the Word in Psychoanalysis
Selected Papers of Pere Folch Mateu
Edited by J.O. Esteve and Jordi Sala

The Freudian Matrix of André Green
Towards a Psychoanalysis for the 21st Century
Edited by Howard B. Levine

Desire, Pain and Thought
Primal Masochism and Psychoanalytic Theory
Marilia Aisenstein

Trauma and Pain Without a Subject
Disruptive Marks in the Psyche, Resignified
Juan-Eduardo Tesone

Outsider Art and Psychoanalytic Psychiatry
The 'Nativity of Fools' at the Cogoleto Psychiatric Hospital
Cosimo Schinaia

The Astonishing Adolescent Upheaval in Psychoanalysis
Edited by Roosevelt Cassorla and Silvia Flechner

The Astonishing Adolescent Upheaval in Psychoanalysis

Edited by
Roosevelt Cassorla and Silvia Flechner

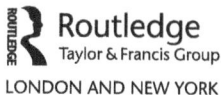
Routledge
Taylor & Francis Group

LONDON AND NEW YORK

Designed cover image: © Getty Images

First published 2024
by Routledge
4 Park Square, Milton Park, Abingdon, Oxon OX14 4RN

and by Routledge
605 Third Avenue, New York, NY 10158

Routledge is an imprint of the Taylor & Francis Group, an informa business

British Library Cataloguing-in-Publication Data
A catalogue record for this book is available from the British Library

Library of Congress Cataloging-in-Publication Data
Names: Cassorla, Roosevelt M. S. (Roosevelt Moises Smeke), editor. | Flechner, Silvia, editor.
Title: The astonishing adolescent upheaval in psychoanalysis / edited by Roosevelt Cassorla and Silvia Flechner.
Description: Abingdon, Oxon ; New York, NY : Routledge, 2024. | Series: Psychoanalytic ideas and applications series | Includes bibliographical references and index. |
Identifiers: LCCN 2023042212 (print) | LCCN 2023042213 (ebook) |
Subjects: LCSH: Adolescent analysis.
Classification: LCC RJ503 .A88 2024 (print) | LCC RJ503 (ebook) | DDC 616.89/170835–dc23/eng/20231213 LC record available at https://lccn.loc.gov/2023042212
LC ebook record available at https://lccn.loc.gov/2023042213

ISBN: 978-1-032-46151-9 (hbk)
ISBN: 978-1-032-46150-2 (pbk)
ISBN: 978-1-003-38028-3 (ebk)

DOI: 10.4324/9781003380283

Typeset in Palatino
by Taylor & Francis Books

Contents

Series foreword

The Publications Committee of the IPA is pleased to present another book in the Psychoanalytic Ideas and Application Series – *The Astonishing Adolescent Upheaval in Psychoanalysis*.

Adolescent psychoanalysis constantly confronts us with a transit process in which life, acting, sexuality, and death are played out. The instinctual (trieb) movements that peculiarly come into play predominantly are expressed through the body as acting out or passage to act; acting that, in many cases, takes the form of an intrusive and violent act for the adolescent himself or for his environment.

The pubescent body and its passage to adolescence is always a complicated moment due to a transformational psychophysical state. The adolescent body can escape self-control and thus harm or attack itself or others. Self-harm, as well as other symptoms, such as drug addiction or anorexia or bulimia nervosa, are some examples of profound disorders that originate in the mother-infant relationship, subsequently being involved in family, social and cultural factors.

The contributions to this book aim to show, from a theoretical-clinical point of view, the enormous difficulties that adolescents go through from a broad point of view and tries to cover the thought of psychoanalysts from different regions, thus showing their peculiarities and characteristics.

We hope that it will be helpful for all those analysts who work with adolescents and that the book opens up new conceptualizations about treatment in the analysis of adolescent patients.

Silvia Flechner
Series Editor
Chair IPA Publications Committee

Foreword

The treatment of adolescent patients will always be a challenge for the analyst. The catastrophic repetition of an original insufficiency in the relationship between the mother and the baby will generate a broad range of situations of extreme danger that will appear throughout childhood but will be defined in adolescence.

Broadly, the kind of difficulties with which adolescents develop nowadays starts from early intrapsychic conflicts. The consequences show pathologies reflected in acting out with high degrees of risk framed within positions, such as addiction, anorexia, aggression, and violence, including death, indicating the impossibility of control of any limit, whether internal or external. Their aggravation allows us to question ourselves about the contemporary adult's psychic libidinal economy, crystallizing unusually during adolescence. What do we see in young adolescents today? First, there would seem to be a lack of interest in sexuality, a desexualizing excitement; motivations are centred much more on extreme situations, addictions of all kinds, including social networks, as a matter of isolation, and events that seem to have more to do with "stopping the feelings" or not being emotionally involved as far as the excitement that can generate a certain subjection with the other.

However, despite the changes, oedipal anxiety is always present. It will appear covert and masked yet in need of understanding. In those cases of early abandonment by the adult, where the absence of the presence of the word, or the limit, becomes the trace of external reality, the adolescent will remain a prisoner of his intrapsychic conflicts that overflow and surpass him, giving way to actions that always carry a deadly connotation. They are in search of a defensive hardening that then becomes more of a lair in which they will try to hide. This attempt to avoid showing actual suffering is linked to a continuing, enormous dependency on the oedipal parents.

For example, threatened by violent drives and by contact with reality, the young person seeks protection in an idealized object. Adherence to this object will be proportional to the feelings of terrifying helplessness that bring back traumas experienced in early life. Clinically speaking, these young people put themselves in symbiosis with an object. By analogy, we can say that the young person becomes addicted to the object, or is "fanatic" for it.

When the configurations become rigid, we come face to face with the functioning of narcissistic pathological organizations.

The triangular reality, however, threatens the preservation of the symbiotic-parasitic relationship. When it is broken, the young person is assaulted by the terrors of annihilation. Hence, the term "fanatic" makes more sense when there is violence against a "betraying" object that has detached itself from the symbiotic self.

Sometimes there is a suicidal act, which, apart from vengeance, seeks an idealized life after death. In situations of intense resentment (triggered, for example, by chronic bullying), the young person may attack their schoolmates with a firearm and subsequently commit suicide. The necessity of a dual relationship is an essential factor contributing to people becoming attached to religious, ideological, mystical, or criminal groups, etc. The idealized object fills the void, and the alleged power of the group is assumed. A person may identify with one truth, which will become their cause. Fanatic groups, such as Nazis, Communists, or other youth groups, are constituted to spearhead the dissemination of the alleged truth.

Deprived children and adolescents involved with criminal organizations begin to feel they "exist." In precarious social situations, it is easier to find weakened persons who, when feeling welcomed, join the relative group and become fanatics. Addiction to dietary systems, physical exercise, drugs, gambling, the internet, work and so on, may reveal similar defensive organizations that persist into adult life. Sometimes society accepts and stimulates this type of "fanaticism." We are dealing with narcissistic organizations that protect against psychotic explosion. However, when the defences falter, the frustrating object becomes threatening and is attacked vengefully and resentfully.

Body changes and space-time changes generate a sense of wonder in the adolescent, a fragile tissue that moulds the body without the psyche accompanying this process. The difficulties caused by this gap can bring, in turn, critical psychopathological consequences that must be addressed promptly, given the characteristics of a psyche that has not yet evolved and matured concerning the acceptance and recognition of such changes.

The chapters in this book aim to account for the clinical realities we face today in treating adolescents with different types of disturbances at the psychic level. One is narcissistic suffering, representing many cures in private practice and psychotherapy treatments in institutions. It proposes a path little explored in the classical clinical literature, in the prolongation of certain intuitions of Freud and D.W. Winnicott, which extends by introducing the project of reconstructing what remains of "narcissistic" and solipsistic propositions in the theories of narcissism.

Our goal consists in attempting to re-establish, whenever necessary, the impact of the responses of significant objects in the impasses present in narcissistic suffering. Based on the hypothesis originating from Freud but still unknown, the dilemmas and paradoxes of subject narcissism arise not only from a "loss of object" or the absence of narcissistic objects, but from their mode of presence and the primary disappointments encountered in the attitude of the existence of these objects.

The texts try to provide much more satisfactory therapeutic results. Intersubjectivity is marked by the importance of moving from parents to group references. It is thus a central prototype of this approach. The theory and clinical orientation given to both theory and practice keep the construction/ reconstruction of history, particularly of the early history of the subject, at the centre of its style.

Roosevelt M. Cassorla
Silvia Flechner

Contributors

Roosevelt Cassorla, MD, PhD, is a training analyst of the Brazilian Psychoanalytic Societies of São Paulo and Campinas. He is Full Professor at the State University of Campinas, collaborator on the IPA Encyclopedic Dictionary and member of the College of *The International Journal of Psychoanalysis*. His previous books are *Advances in Contemporary Psychoanalytic Field Theory*, co-edited with M. Katz and G. Civitarese (Routledge), *The Psychoanalyst, the Theatre of Dreams and the Clinic of Enactment* (Routledge) and *Studies on Suicide: Psychoanalysis and Mental Health* (in Portuguese, Blucher). He received the 2017 Mary S. Sigourney Award for Outstanding Achievement in Psychoanalysis.

Silvia Flechner, MD, is a child, adolescent, and adult training analyst of the Uruguayan Psychoanalytical Society, a psychologist, and Master in Psychoanalysis. She was the Publications Committee Chair (2021–2025); International New Groups (ING) IPA Co-Chair for Latin America (2018–2021); former President and former Scientific Director of the Uruguayan Psychoanalytic Association; past Director of the master's degree in psychoanalysis for candidates of the Institute of Psychoanalysis issued by the Universidad de la República Del Uruguay. She was also a former director of the Board of the Training Committee; member of the Assessor and Organizing Committee as co/editor for the "International Journal Conference" in Rio de Janeiro (2004). She was the winner of the Child and Adolescent prize in the FEPAL Congress, Santiago de Chile (2008). Flechner has been a reviewer and member of the Board of the *International Journal of Psychoanalysis* since 2008. Teaching seminars in Montevideo, invited teachers from Latin American countries, she has also published papers in the *International Journal of Psychoanalysis* and numerous journals in Latin America and other countries. Compiler and contributor to *Psicoanálisis y adolescencia: dos temporalidades que se interpelan* (Psicolibro Ediciones, Librería Paidos, Buenos Aires); co/editor of *Truth, Reality and the Psychoanalyst*, edited by the Publications Committee of the IPA (in English and Spanish), she was also in charge of the edition and press of the Spanish version in Uruguay (2005).

Martin Gauthier MD, is a child and adolescent psychiatrist and a training analyst in private practice in Montreal. For 35 years, he worked with children and adolescents at the Montreal Children's Hospital and taught at McGill University. He is a former President of the Canadian Psychoanalytic Society and of the Société psychanalytique de Montréal, as well as a former North American representative on the Board of the International Psychoanalytic Association. He has presented and published in various psychoanalytic conferences and journals.

Virginia Ungar MD, is a training analyst at the Buenos Aires Psychoanalytic Association. She has taught at the Institute of Psychoanalysis and in other societies in Argentina and abroad such as Brazil, Chile, the US and Europe. She has published numerous articles in psychoanalytic journals and book chapters. She was the former Chair of the IPA's Child and Adolescent Psychoanalysis Committee (COCAP) and of the Committee for Integrated Training. In 2016, she was awarded the Platinum Konex Award, for the most outstanding personality of the last decade in the discipline of psychoanalysis. She is the former President of the IPA (2017–2021), the first woman to be elected to that position since the IPA's inception.

François Ladame MD is past Professor of Psychiatry at the University of Geneva and Chair of the Units for Adolescents and Young Adults and is currently working as a psychoanalyst in private practice in Geneva. A past President and training analyst of the Swiss Psychoanalytical Society; European Psychoanalytic Federation: Past Chair of the Nomination Committee and past Member of the House Committee, co-founder of the Forum on Adolescence. For the International Psychoanalytical Association: member of the former House of Delegates and past European representative to the Board; past Chair of the Sponsoring Committee to the Lebanese study group. He has published 40 book chapters and more than a hundred scientific papers.

Carlos Moguillansky MD and Master in Sociology of Culture (UNSAM), is a trainer and supervising psychoanalyst of the Buenos Aires Psychoanalytic Association, IPA. Former Scientific Secretary and President of APDEBA. During his presidency, the IUSAM Mental Health Institute was founded and the first IPA psychoanalytic university institute in Latin America. He is a faculty member of the University of Buenos Aires (UBA), USAL and IUSAM and invited Professor in Mexico, Panama and Brazil. He is a former member of the Board of *The International Journal of Psychoanalysis* and current member of the IPA Publications Committee. He is the author of numerous papers in Argentina and foreign magazines and of the books *Adolescent Clinic, Latencies, Saying the Impossible* and *Pain and its Defences*. He has participated as author and editor in numerous anthologies in Spanish and English.

Mary Brady, PhD, is an adult and child psychoanalyst in private practice in San Francisco. She is on the faculty of the San Francisco Center for Psychoanalysis. Her book, *The Body in Adolescence: Psychic Isolation and Physical Symptoms* was published by Routledge in 2016. In it she discusses the relationship of psychic isolation, along with other factors, to physical expressions which emerge during adolescence, including eating disorders, cutting, substance abuse and suicide attempts. Her recent book, *Analytic Engagements with Adolescents: Sex, Gender and Subversion,* was published by Routledge in 2018. In this book she discusses the distinctiveness of adolescent treatment in its 'heat' and intensity. Adolescents and their analysts experience this intensity in various ways. Enormous bodily change, subversiveness and rebellion against authority, parental response, and family dynamics, all enliven and sometimes threaten to overwhelm the analytic relationship.

Ruggero Levy, psychoanalyst, effective member and training analyst of the Psychoanalytic Society of Porto Alegre and of the IPA, former President of SPPA; co-chair for Latin America of the Program Committee of the 53rd IPA Congress, July 2023, Cartagena, Colombia. Member of the IPA Board 2011–2013 and 2013–2015; Chair of the IPA Working Parties Committee 2017–2021. Author of keynote paper given at the IPA Congress, Buenos Aires in 2017. Professor and supervisor of the Centro de Studos Luiz Guedes, UFRGS and the Center for Studies, Care and Research of Childhood and Adolescence (CEAPIA). Ruggero Levy is the author of several book chapters and scientific articles published in regional, national and international specialized journals, as well as rapporteur and speaker in several national and international scientific events.

Michele Ain is a psychologist and psychoanalyst, Master in Psychoanalysis, and full member of the Uruguayan Psychoanalytic Association. Secretary's President of the Uruguayan Psychoanalytic Association (2012–2014), Chair of the Publications Committee of the Uruguayan Psychoanalytic Association (2016–2018). Publications Committee member IPA (2017–2021); presenter of seminars in child and adolescence, Guadalajara, Mexico.

Nergis Güleç MA, is an IPA adult, child and adolescent psychoanalyst, working in private practice in Istanbul. She is currently the president of IPD (Istanbul Psychoanalytical Association). She is one of the founding and former board members of the İstanbul Child and Adolescent Psychoanalytical Psychotherapy Association (İCEPPD) which is affiliated with EFPP (European Federation for Psychoanalytical Psychotherapy Training, Child and Adolescent section). She is an EFPP accredited Child and Adolescent Psychoanalytical Psychotherapist. She was the IPSO (International Psychoanalytical Studies Organization) Vice President for Europe (2015–2019). She is a member of the IPA Publishing Committee and co-editor of the book *Bebeği Anlamak: Ailesi içinde bebeği gözlemlemek* [Understanding the Baby: Observation of the Infant in the Family] published by Bağlam in 2016.

Thomas Marcacci is a child, adolescent and adult psychoanalyst in private practice in Bologna and full member of the IPA. He is a teacher at the Centro Studi Martha Harris in Bologna. He was editor of the International Psychoanalytical Studies Organization and is part of the IPA Publication Committee. In 2017, he opened a psychoanalytical clinic in Bologna, Centro Evo, where he coordinates a team of psychoanalysts, psychiatrists and educators, working with individuals as well as in community interventions.

1 Stupidity in the analytic field

Vicissitudes of the detachment process in adolescence[1]

Roosevelt M. Cassorla

Over the course of adolescence, the young person feels assailed by drives which reactivate unconscious fantasies and primitive anxieties. The adolescent experiences the rupture of the rigidity of the latency phase, followed by identity confusion resulting from the re-emergence of aspects split off from the self which pertain to the pregenital and preoedipal phases. The enhancement of sadistic aspects in all areas, associated with confusion arising from the concomitance of various fantasies, induces waves of genital desire in all its infantile, polymorphic and perverse forms (Meltzer, 1973, 1992; Grinberg, 1976). The need for immediate gratification produces violent and intrusive projective identifications. Threats of self-dissolution merge with attempts to restructure the self. Primitive and more highly evolved mechanisms also merge, with as much potential to constitute a basis for pathologies as to accommodate elements for redevelopment.

Intrapsychic turbulence is manifested in the stimulation of the PS <-> D oscillation (Bion, 1962) or in that of dual relationships <-> triangular relationships, with the resulting catastrophic changes, yet in a dynamic form, with dissolutions that may confuse the inattentive observer who could interpret a movement which is in fact an intense, yet normal, prefigurement to restructuring to be a pathology. A lack of adequate oscillation will put the analyst on his guard. But it is only once the adolescent turbulence ceases that we will be able to ascertain whether the rigidity was temporary or permanent.

At the same time, externalization and internalization processes intensify to produce conflicts of identification, resulting in an increased vulnerability to the introjection of objects which can reinforce or alter more archaic identifications. The young person is eager for objects to identify with so as to construct a more cohesive adult identity. The projection-introjection interplay is intense; it is precisely the acquisition of an adult identity by means of this interplay of identifications that is considered to be the primary function of adolescence.

The outcome of these configurations leads to movements of detachment, leaving the symbiosis of the family unit (Blos, 1962, Bleger, 1967, Mahler, 1968, Paz, 1980). At the same time, the adolescent experiences mourning: for childhood, parents, the infantile body, and bisexuality (Aberastury, 1980).

DOI: 10.4324/9781003380283-1

If contact with the triangular reality is experienced as traumatic, narcissistic defences are readopted to constitute normal symbioses (Cassorla, 1985, 1991a) until they are overpowered by conflicting drives and attraction for the object. This is part of the development of detachment.

During this period of development links are formed with substitutive objects such as ideals, friends, boy/girlfriends, and idealized parents. This idealization diminishes as the adult identity is established. Yet certain adolescents can settle into a kind of symbiosis or pathological parasitism with these objects. In the clinic, this sense of being held captive by the object can manifest itself as addictive behaviours involving people, groups, drugs, ideologies, and religious sects, as suicidal acts (when the patient has fantasies of an idealized life in another world), and as teenage pregnancy (when the young woman becomes symbiotic with her baby). The capacity for symbolization is blocked. In other cases, the young person may become prematurely independent (Cassorla, 1985, 1991a) in a manic reaction against the desire for symbiosis. Those who prolong their adolescence into later years, referred to as "adultescents" (Ungar, 2013), also belong in this category.

The analytic experience with these young patients can bring the analyst into contact with challenging situations, due to defensive organizations which prove difficult to access (Cassorla, 1997a, 2001, 2004, 2005). These organizations can draw in people close to the patient's family, which may also include the analyst. The latter may allow himself to be drawn into the organization without fully realizing it. This gives the external observer the impression that a numbed analytic capacity has led the analyst to become *stupid* (Bion, 1967).

Objectives

The objective of this chapter is to deepen the understanding of the technical vicissitudes that emerge in the face of defensive organizations, which protect adolescent patients from contact with the triangular reality. It will specifically address the ways in which these aspects are manifested in the analytic field, the factors that draw the analyst into the defensive organization, the origins and consequences of his numbed perception or stupidity, and the factors related to dealing with family members who participate in these organizations. Both clinical material and material from myths of adolescent heroes will be drawn upon to achieve this.

Stupidity in the myths of Narcissus and Oedipus

The analyst's possible stupidity when working with adolescents can reflect a similar numbed perception on the part of the young person, which occurs during the detachment process. Mythical narratives can serve as models to illustrate this phenomenon. Studying these enables us to identify two complementary senses of the term stupidity, which will prove useful in the clinic.

First, in the myth of Narcissus the eponymous character falls in love with his own image reflected in the waters of a lake. Narcissus' inability to discern self from object reveals his numbed perception. In one version of the myth this stupidity results in Narcissus drowning in an attempt to reach the idealized object, which he does not realize to be his own reflection.

Transposing this situation into the analytic field, we find ourselves in an area in which analyst and patient establish a fusional relationship through cross-identifications. Each feels the other to be an extension of their respective self. They may both be unaware that this is happening. When this occurs the analytic process remains frozen in the dual area of fusion-confusion, even while development may proceed in other areas.

Second, another sense of the term 'stupidity' refers to the impossibility of Narcissus accepting the love of Echo the nymph. We can consider Narcissus' rejection to be a result of his terror of coming into contact with the self/object differentiation. Thus the function of stupidity is to avoid contact with the triangular reality in seeking to maintain the fantasy of narcissistic completion.

The transposition of this second sense into the analytic field reveals situations in which the perception of the triangular reality is attacked. The threat of self/object differentiation triggers catastrophic anxiety, which is discharged at the same time as the analytic dyad returns to the fusional situation. When the patient (rightly) attributes this perception to the analytic work, this work will be attacked. The analyst's thinking capacity is blocked by massive projective identifications. These can latch onto the professional's personal qualities. Therefore, both the re-establishment of the dual relationship and the stupidity are preceded by the unbearable glimmer of contact with reality.

The Oedipus myth reveals situations to complement that of Narcissus. If the latter's initial state is one of undifferentiated fusion, with the triangular reality as threat, in the oedipal myth the acquired triangularity is what becomes dangerous. For this reason it is reversed. This occurs, for example, when Sophocles (in *Oedipus Rex*) describes the beginning of Oedipus's investigation in the search for Laius's murderer. As he is consulting Tiresias, they have a tense and aggressive exchange in which Tiresias "opens Oedipus's eyes". Oedipus defends himself from the threatening perception, accusing Tiresias of colluding with Creon (Jocasta's brother) to steal the throne from him. The projection of voracious and envious aspects within the Tiresias-Creon dyad liberates the Oedipus-Jocasta dyad; the true usurpers of Laius's throne.[2]

The configurations implied in these two senses of the term stupidity oscillate in a double meaning: frozen dual relationship <-> threat of perception of the triangular reality. Stupidity therefore manifests itself in two ways: 1. The impossibility of the dual relationship to perceive itself; 2. The impossibility of experiencing the triangular reality.

The models described relate to working with patients who present difficulties with perceiving and living in the triangular reality where self and object are distinct from one another. Of these patients, there are some for whom borderline configurations predominate, that is, where parts which were split off live in a world of dual relationships while others maintain contact with the triangular reality. These patients have been unable to develop oedipal situations in certain areas of their minds, and thus either return to or remain in narcissistic situations. On the other hand, attraction to narcissistic situations can reveal traumas that make this development difficult.

If we acknowledge that myths can describe emotional configurations, it should come as no surprise to us that Narcissus and Oedipus are adolescents. For it is precisely during adolescence that the oscillation and confusion between narcissistic and oedipal aspects come to the fore with such intensity. When these aspects are insufficiently developed they can form stable, defensive organizations.

Let us remember that Narcissus and Oedipus coexist within the same adolescent individual, and the oscillation between dual and triangular relationships reveals the same oscillation between PS<->D. On the border between these two configurations, the young person resembles Hamlet: "To be or not to be, that is the question." "Not to be" is manifested as narcissistic collusion and mortiferous undifferentiation, and "to be" as the unbearable contact with reality (Cassorla, 1997b, 2009).

The clinic[3]

I know that I am annoyed with Katia. I also know that I am feeling worried and powerless. This is the fourth session in a row that Katia has missed. In the previous instances, her father's secretary would usually leave a voice message. "Katia asked me to let you know that she will be unable to attend because …". The reason was clarified: "she had to travel with her mother", "she has a doctor's appointment", "she's gone out with her father …"

Despite feeling annoyed by these messages, and by the secretary's role as intermediary between us, I felt a certain change – some consideration for me as a person. Before, Katia would scarcely bother to warn me. She missed many sessions and when she eventually did appear she behaved as if nothing had happened. When I investigated factors relating to the sessions missed, Katia would say, as if it were obvious, that she had been absent due to another engagement. As far as Katia was concerned there was no reason to inform her analyst, either before or after her absence. The analytic investigation became blocked.

Katia had begun analysis with me a few months earlier. In the first few sessions, she reticently conveyed to me facts indicative of a psychotic break; the most evident manifestation of which took place two years previously when she had moved to study in the city of H. She was 17 years old at the time. When she moved to H, Katia had recently stopped attending therapy, which she had started aged 7. She told me how after a while her therapist also began to treat her mother, her sister, and for a time her father, on separate schedules. When the therapist began to "badmouth" her parents and demanded secrecy, Katia became confused. After a few weeks she related the incident to her parents and they all ceased their treatment. This information, or fantasies of Katia's, made me suspect the intensity of the crossed projective identifications in this family unit. It also helped me to formulate hypotheses on the source of the unease I had experienced at the beginning of the analysis. The first interview was arranged by her mother, who told me over the phone that her parents would prefer not to speak with me and that I should engage directly with Katia. This apparent respect for her individuality pleasantly surprised me.

Nonetheless, after the first few sessions in which I felt confused about certain pieces of information, I resolved to speak with her parents. Katia told me emphatically that she did not want me to talk to them. She did not know how to tell me what her reasons were and I noticed that she did not admit to continuing to investigate the issue. I imagined that if I failed to respect her request she would no longer confide in me. On the other hand, I felt safe in the knowledge that Katia was consulting a psychiatrist whom I trusted.

Unbeknownst to me, I was already involved in a sadomasochistic collusion in which I was paralysed by both Katia and her parents. My initial idealization of the family's respect for her individuality had transformed into a sub-mission to their desires. For a while I maintained this idealization without fully realizing the submission. I had become stupid and blind, despite the fact that in other areas of my mind I suspected that something was wrong. At a later date I was to discover that the family had denied me access to certain pieces of information so as to protect itself from the potential detachment of one of its members.

It soon became clear to me that Katia's psychotic aspects were persisting and that her diffidence was designed to conceal them, while also signalling their presence. The sessions always began with the line, "I'm fine, getting better" followed by "That's all" and "Nothing else to say". Her silence prompted me to start a conversation and I would ask her questions. Katia's monosyllabic responses could exasperate me, and I had to take care not to force the investigation. On some occasions it seemed like Katia, as if feeling sorry for me, would be about to tell me something else but as soon as I went to investigate, her account abruptly halted. Katia felt that my participation in her life was very dangerous. Sometimes she came closer, with great caution, but my correspondence made her retreat again. When I tried to show Katia these movements she ignored me. Despite feeling powerless and confused I believed that if I continued patiently with my work things would become clearer in time. I behaved like the waiter at the "bar in the desert" (Bolognini, 2004) who greets the guest in the way that she presents herself.

By trying to convince me that she was "getting better" Katia was attempting to draw me into an idealized collusion. On other occasions she would provide promising information that did not strike me as truthful. At the same time, it was not difficult to perceive the attacks on the analytic process that manifested themselves as absences, reticence in recounting events, and delays in payment. But noticing these was not enough to broaden thinking capacity. Later, I was to realize that I was partially involved in dual collusions.

Katia was gradually able to provide me with details about the psychotic break accompanied by rationalized explanations. It was a phase in which "I felt like I was in unity with God and the Universe". She felt nostalgic for this time and would like to return. But at the same time she lived in terror. On one occasion she ran out into the streets with no destination and was helped by the police. She believed that her episodes were caused by witchcraft, by drugs her friends had made her ingest without her knowledge. And they would have done this because they were jealous of her boyfriend and her intellect.

It was possible to observe that her predominant relationships at the time of the break were idealized symbiotic relations with female friends and with her boyfriend, alternating or becoming confused with sadomasochistic relations involving violence, blackmail, submissions and seductions. Sexuality was also revealed to be confused.

Katia conveyed to me an image of her parents as heirs of the lineage of a great noble family. They believed they were descendants of a certain European royal family. This highlighted the supposed blindness of the parents who believed Katia was merely "stressed". The theory of poisoning through drugs seemed to have been conveniently sustained by everyone.

Katia's monotonous and controlled speech, characterized by blunted affect, imprisoned the analytic process and revealed the prison in which she lived. The few things she did recount related to the past. Katia disregarded any statement pertaining to the present and to what was happening in the analytic field.

Katia told me how, during the psychotic break, she had begun analysis in the city of H. After some weeks the analyst warned the family, without her knowledge, that Katia was psychotic. The information must have shaken the family pride and analysis was stopped. Strangely, the family seemed to ignore the fact that she was taking antipsychotic medication at the time.

The expressive way in which Katia told me about the "unethical behaviour" of the analyst (this time without any blunted affect on her part) confused me, and I began to imagine the analyst to have been inadequate. I quickly realized that I had been recruited to take her side against the therapist. The dullness of my analytic capacity led me to make moralistic evaluations of what had occurred "outside and in the past", leaving me virtually blind to the "here and now". I soon realized the obvious: that Katia was warning me of the risks I would be running if I confronted her with the madness. The symbiotic Royal Family would come to the rescue of the Princess in distress.

I gradually discovered that before moving city Katia had been a "good-natured and obedient" girl. Given the hypothesis that Katia was trying to extract herself from the symbiosis with her parents, the experience of moving to H became clear. The sudden contact with the triangular reality manifested itself as a psychotic break, revealing the terror of annihilation as a consequence of the detachment experienced as traumatic. To avoid coming into contact with this trauma in the analytic field, the "good-natured" pseudo-mature girl (Meltzer, 1966) and her perfect family recruited me to participate in the family symbiosis. Their arsenal of powerful weapons included massive projective identification which could block my perception of the facts by rendering me stupid.

Undoing collusions

After nearly a year of analysis Katia committed a slip of the tongue and from this I discovered that she had been concealing an important decision from me; one which had significantly altered her life. When questioned on the reason for her omission she provided a weak excuse. I felt disregarded and deceived.

On this occasion, trying consciously to control my anger, I warned Katia that if she continued to omit information it would make the analysis impossible. I tried to speak calmly. While I was talking I felt worried, certain that Katia had noticed my irritation. I imagined that I was losing the analytic vertex and functioning as a morally condemnatory superego. As Katia continued to receive me with indifference, my confusion grew and I became certain of my stupidity.

I expected Katia to become resentful of my observations. However, after this incident the analysis acquired some surprising new aspects. Katia no longer missed sessions. Her spoken accounts were more symbolic. In this period it became increasingly clear to me that a large part of the material that she had presented (and concealed) during the previous phase of analysis had been composed either of elements without meaning, or of deteriorated symbols (Cassorla, 2013a, 2013b) which had lost their expressive function (Barros, 2011).

I gradually realized that, along with her collaborative side, Katia was subtly revealing another side to her which was exaggeratedly "good-natured". I noticed how she seductively tried to immobilize me. This fact alerted me to the possibility of a subsequent catastrophic rupture. In this phase, Katia seemed to notice the vicissitudes of the oscillation between the dual relationship and the terrible consequences resulting from her perception of differentiation from the other, but only outside the analytic field. She behaved in a controlling manner towards friends and boyfriends and reacted to fantasies or threats of rupture with violence, blackmail, and victimization. At certain moments, faced with Katia's despair and her terror of non-existence, I imagined she could become self-destructive or make some gesture of suicide. My intuition was revealed to be correct when she suffered an accident while driving under the influence of alcohol on a public holiday, when I had extended my holidays. Katia, however, was not in a condition to consider the feelings that would arise in the analytic field.

A few weeks later Katia reverted to missing sessions again, this time with no advance warning. After three consecutive absences I telephoned her household. The secretary informed me that Katia was sleeping. I asked for Katia to call me. Nothing happened. The absences continued. I telephoned again and after multiple attempts I managed to get through to the secretary. She spontaneously told me that Katia was behaving strangely, locking herself in her room and hardly speaking. She expressed sympathy for me with regard to Katia missing the analysis sessions and imagined that I must be concerned. I viewed the secretary as a part of the Royal Family, albeit more distinct from the rest of them. This perception encouraged me to question her about Katia's parents. The secretary informed me that they were travelling, having left some weeks ago "now that the lady is better". I left the conversation in the knowledge that the lady, Katia's mother, suffered from a serious, life-threatening illness. I felt irritated with Katia for not having told me. I saw myself reformulating the whole prior analytic process in my mind. I asked for the parents to telephone me as soon as they returned from their trip, despite my awareness that Katia did not want me to talk to them.

Katia continued to ignore my messages. I imagined she could be experiencing a psychotic break and may have been at risk of suicide. I was in anguish without any kind of hypothesis on what was happening. During this period a scientific event was taking place in another city. I could not stop thinking about Katia and I felt inappropriate when discussing the situation with a kind colleague whom I barely knew. I was searching for auxiliary dreamers for something I myself was unable to symbolize.

Katia's mother called me days later, surprised that Katia was missing her sessions. I arranged an interview with the parents. But before this took place, Katia returned to her habitual schedule. She told me that she was fine. She had been absent because she was very busy. She knew that I wished to speak with her parents and she wanted to know my reasons. I told her there were things that remained unclear which her parents might be able to clarify for me. I made it clear that I would not be dissuaded from meeting with them. I was trying to investigate factors related to her absences and I informed her that her excuse, claiming she had been very busy, made little sense to me.

At that moment Katia announced, angrily, that she had turned up to a session but that I had not been there. I discovered that this had happened on a day when Katia would have been my first patient, because the patient before her was not coming. I remembered that I had arrived five minutes before her scheduled appointment time and had been relieved to find that I had arrived before her. Katia had in fact arrived slightly before me but, on seeing the clinic closed, she left. I asked her why she did not wait for me. She said that since I was not expecting her, she had concluded that I did not want to treat her anymore.

It was possible to use this episode to demonstrate to Katia her anger at having felt rejected. This was why she had abandoned me. Katia had projected onto me the terror of annihilation she experienced when faced with the perception that I was another person with my own life. During our conversation I put forward a model. Like a servant, I should be ever ready to anticipate the princess's needs and desires. Because I had not behaved correctly, the princess had expelled me. By ignoring my existence she was behaving so as to make me feel the terror of non-existence that she experienced constantly, but she could not be clear on this. (In not knowing how to symbolize it and dream it, this annihilating non-existence was experienced terrifyingly as a thing-in-itself). At the same time Katia expected that I, despairing over the experience of non-existence, would find her and apologize. My messages, however, had been ignored because her resentment prevented her from relenting.

During these interpretations Katia referred to the relationship with her boyfriend. She was aware that she projected her own helplessness onto him, along with the vital need to be seen and noticed. Katia associated this repetitive compulsion with what was taking place in the analytic field. Now, the analytic dyad could dream-for-two. At one point, when I remarked that it seemed as though I was more interested in her analysis than she was, Katia laughed openly in a way that I had never seen her do before, and I found myself laughing with her.

My analytic function was re-established. The presence of the third person (the servant who was not a servant, and was therefore not waiting on the princess) and the possibility of discussing this issue, dreaming it together, showed the dual relationship being undone.

This episode, together with the one described earlier in which I angrily brought the omission of information to Katia's attention, reveals another kind of stupidity in the analytic field. It relates to acute enactments, which undo the chronic collusions. The study of these concepts will begin below.

The next session validated the work done beforehand when Katia brought me the account of a dream; something she had never done before. She was attacked by a group of savages. She sensed they were about to open fire on her. Their guns were lipsticks and the bullets were sweets. She managed to dodge the bullets. It was terrifying, but the best part was when she woke up and realized it was only a dream. She told me that it was one of the best sensations of her life. I showed her how she was now able to dream at night about the terrors that used to haunt her 24 hours a day. Katia's dream revealed the presence of a contact-barrier (Bion, 1962) which was formed at the same time as the emergence of the capacity for symbolization and the work through of the oedipal situation. In her dream, Katia was trying to give meaning to areas of violence and sexuality.

During our conversation about her mother's illness (information she had previously omitted) Katia showed how she had been trying to deny it. She protected herself from the terror of losing her, and from the guilt of having abandoned her, by moving to H. The illness had emerged soon after her move. Possibilities were opened up for our future collaboration, working on reliving her attacks, feelings of guilt, and oedipal retaliations.

The meeting with her parents took place after multiple cancellations on their part. Katia did not want to participate. Her parents were second cousins and their families had lived together for generations. The information they provided made me strongly suspect the transgenerational transmission of symbiotic defences. Her parents decided that they would rather not see me, so as to avoid problems caused by the "gossip" from other therapists. Oscillating towards the other extreme, they were also controlling me through lack of information. In this way they were attempting to maintain the family symbiosis. It was also possible to observe that this had been an appropriate time to interview these parents.

During our conversation the parents eventually admitted that their daughter had experienced a psychotic break and they thought it might happen again at any moment. They confessed their fear since mental illness was already in the family; it was a family secret. They were also aware that the mother's illness had shaken the integration (in fact, the symbiosis) of the family. The prognosis for the mother's illness, formerly terrible, had now improved. They were beginning family therapy. I cautiously suggested that they might also consider individual treatment … with different analysts …

Returning to technical aspects

The clinical situation I have described demonstrates how oscillations between narcissistic and oedipal configurations are manifested in the analytic field. Katia's detachment process was disturbed due to archaic identifications with objects in symbiosis, which became the basis for narcissistic refuges whose potential rupture led to psychotic decompensation.

When dealing with patients with these characteristics, the psychoanalyst runs the risks highlighted in the myths studied earlier. Patient and analyst can form mutual idealization collusions, like Narcissus and his reflection in the lake. Collusions of domination/submission can occur when the analyst assumes the role of Echo, seeking to prise the patient from their narcissistic refuge.

The idealized collusion can be rapidly transformed into a sadomasochistic collusion, and vice-versa. Since the idealization cannot be permanently maintained, the patient becomes resentful and starts attacking the analyst who can either submit or retaliate, and the patient responds in turn. Manic reparations make it oscillate back to idealization, and so it continues.

Phenomenologically speaking, the oscillation between idealized and sadomasochistic collusions manifests itself in the form of seductions and attacks such as blackmail, victimization, self-destructive acts etc., which persist in a resentful form. These situations are a constant feature of working with adolescents.

As we have seen, clinical work with adolescents requires some knowledge of the relationship, both real and internalized, with the parents. In the myths of Narcissus and Oedipus there are indications of idealized relationships with mothers. It is possible to imagine Liriope falling in love with her beautiful son Narcissus while drawing him away from the triangular reality. Jocasta, in turn, "closes her eyes" to the perception that Oedipus could be her son and helps him to conquer the paternal throne.[4]

The events described above alert us to the network of crossed projective identifications that occupies the analytic field when we work with adolescents. These can involve parents, family members, teachers, romantic partners; adolescents may also try to recruit the analyst. The analyst cannot refrain from necessary conversation with family members. Generally, the patient does not wish to participate in these meetings, as though intuiting the parents' need for their own space. The analyst will also have to "listen out" for his own internal aspects which may be identified with the adolescent's parents.

Vicissitudes relating to the collusion between patient and analyst have been discussed by various authors. Possibly the first collusion relating to psychoanalysis occurred between Breuer and Anna O., which culminated in the interruption of treatment (Freud, 1893). Freud (1905) writes of his numbed perception with Dora, which leads him to intuit the phenomenon of transference. In neither case did they sufficiently realize their own involvement, whether romantic or destructive. Winnicott (1949) indicates that in certain situations the analyst needs to somehow demonstrate the anger that the patient has induced in him. Otherwise the patient will not believe that they can induce love. The manifestation of anger can undo dual collusions, as in Katia's case, even when the analyst appears stupid. It is clear that the situations will have to be recognized and developed in order for them to become useful.

Bion (1967) demonstrated that the presence of the *stupidity, arrogance and curiosity* triad in the analytic field simultaneously conceals and reveals destructive psychological catastrophe. The stupidity we have reflected on in the collusions studied is accompanied by the other components of the triad.

The patient manifests *curiosity* by wishing to continue their analysis, insufficiently aware of their desire to fuse with the analyst. The analyst frustrates the patient if he maintains his own mind and does not allow anybody to fuse with him. When the dual relationship is undone, the patient feels expelled from the dual "paradise" in having to confront the traumatic triangular reality.[5]

Arrogance is linked to omniscience and to the moralistic evaluation that substitutes the perception of reality with condemnatory judgement. Any information that points to the existence of the other, the triangular reality, will be omnisciently considered to be bad or wrong. The patient dictatorially condemns anything that threatens the dual relationship. What the observer perceives to be arrogance, the patient perceives to be the legitimate exercise of their rights.

Stupidity is linked to deficiencies in the capacity for symbolization, dreaming, and thinking. As we have seen, it can be manifested as omniscience, dual collusions, and/or as discharges in the face of contact with the triangular reality. The distortion of reality and the condemnatory vision of the frustrating force link stupidity with arrogance.

As we have seen, the analyst runs the risk of being recruited and *becoming* an aspect of the psychotic part of the patient. With adolescents, this recruitment is made possible through crossed projective identifications, which draw other people in who are close to the young person. The analyst identifies with the arrogance and stupidity that form part of the family symbiosis. The analyst can also become a depository for persecutory and depressive feelings of guilt when he imagines that he is traumatizing the patient and their family by revealing the triangular reality to them.

Bion (1961) describes similar situations in studying groups. The analyst does not notice that his mind is in a state of torpor and that he is accepting as reality what is in fact a product of massive projective identifications. The analyst imagines the intense feelings that he experiences to be entirely justified by the objective situation. Subsequently, Bion would attribute this torpor to the action of the beta screen which provokes in the analyst what the patient desires. Analysts, supervisors, and groups of analysts can jointly maintain this mental torpor (Cassorla, 2013c).

Joseph (1989) elegantly demonstrates how the analyst is recruited to represent aspects of the patient in order to maintain the status quo. Besides Bion and Joseph, other pioneering authors in the study of massive projective identifications include Grinberg, Rosenfeld, Sandler, Grotstein, Ogden, etc., who also study how the analyst is recruited and induced to become an aspect of the patient, a subject already suggested by Ferenczi.[6]

The self-perception of stupidity on the analyst's part may never be achieved, resulting in paralysis in the field in the area in question, and in analytic impasses. The stupidity may be perceived when the analyst discusses his material with colleagues or when he writes about or reflects upon his sense of unease, taking a second look (Baranger, Baranger & Mom, 1983) or by listening to listening (Faimberg, 1996). And yet, as we have seen from the clinical material, stupidity can be perceived, apparently paradoxically, when it is revealed in the second sense of the term that we studied, in other words when there is a threat of rupture in the analytic field. This fact prompts the analyst to investigate. Consequently, that is, *après-coup*, the analyst realizes his prior stupidity in relation to the dual collusions.

On enactments

Certain ideas about enactment can help us to understand the situations described. The mutual recruitments which maintain the dual relationship have been called *chronic enactments*. The adolescent, fearing detachment, protects herself from the perception of the triangular reality. This situation is made possible by symbiotic families in which differentiation between family members is experienced as traumatic. The analyst is also recruited to participate in this symbiosis.

As the capacity for symbolization is re-established, the dual relationship is undone and the triangular relation suddenly appears in the analytic field.

This event has been referred to as *acute enactment*. The analytic dyad (and symbiotic family) lives through the trauma of contact with reality, but in a diminished way. It has been demonstrated that in dual collusions the analyst implicitly exercises the alpha function in parallel areas, mending the ruptures caused by trauma. Once sufficiently repaired, the trauma is relived as it is simultaneously symbolized. As a result, it manifests itself in manageable form. Acute enactment is a mixture of this discharge, the symbolization of elements, and symbolic networks being attacked.

When the acute enactment is induced, the analyst "opens his eyes" to what is happening. At this moment he gains awareness of his former numbed perception, which had prevented him from correctly perceiving the chronic enactments in which he was involved.[7]

Let us return to the clinical material. Initially, Katia, her family, and the analyst were involved in an idealized collusion alternating with a sadomasochistic component. The analyst's initial idealization of her family (with his impression that they respected Katia's individuality) was substituted by a submission to the lack of information. At the same time Katia missed sessions, arrived late, omitted facts, and prevented the analyst from entering into contact with concealed areas. The analyst had a certain degree of awareness of the facts, but this proved insufficient.

This chronic enactment was undone when the analyst gained awareness, as a result of Katia's slip of the tongue, of his own feelings regarding the omission of information. The sequence of facts constituting the first acute enactment studied takes the following form: Katia's omission of information, her revelatory slip, the analyst's anger, his possibly irritated speech, Katia's silence, the analyst's perplexity. This situation, in being signified, connects to the symbolic thought network. Patient and analyst are able to dream-for-two and their thinking capacity broadens over subsequent sessions. But the dual relationship – chronic enactment – is re-established after a few weeks.

The second acute enactment occurs when Katia arrives before her analyst does, and then leaves. The sequence of events takes the following form: Katia arrived at the session early to find her analyst was not there, she felt abandoned and left, the analyst arrived five minutes before the session was due to start and was relieved to find that Katia had not arrived (only weeks later was he to discover that Katia had arrived and left already), the analyst waited for Katia, who did not arrive and continued to be persistently absent for multiple sessions. Katia's idealization of the analyst constantly waiting for her was undone. The resentment re-established the chronic enactment, now in sadomasochistic form, without the acute enactment having been utilized. Her realization would occur weeks later, after the analyst had learned of her mother's illness and demanded to see her parents. Katia returned to analysis before this happened. The analyst's conduct, in calling the parents, could be considered another acute enactment; one which undoes the family symbiosis, at least for the duration of their meeting.

In the situations studied, the two types of dual collusions, sadomasochistic and idealized, occur simultaneously and predominate at certain times. The sadomasochistic type predominates when confronted with defensive config- urations (Steiner, 1993) of the "thick-skinned" kind (Rosenfeld, 1987); in other words, when the adolescent tries to move away from the object in search of a narcissistic refuge (Levy, 1996). This distancing alternates with the search for an idealized collusion. At this moment the configurations are revealed to be "thin-skinned". Sensitivity to the frustration makes the con- figuration revert to "thick-skinned", and so it continues.

Now we have more information to help us understand why in the first epi- sode the analyst had become preoccupied with bringing Katia's omissions to her attention. The analyst intuited that he was undoing the dual relationship and feared that the contact with the triangular situation would be traumatic. At the same time the analyst felt that he could be acting in retaliation towards Katia for her attacks, and felt guilty. This guilt was made possible by his impression of having lost his analytic function. In the second enactment, the analyst's relief to find that he had arrived before Katia reveals intuitions relating to an assumed re-traumatization resulting from the abandonment, and the consequent violent differentiation of self and object.

Reviewing the facts studied, the analyst becomes conscious that he had undergone two reversals of perspective: First, during the chronic enactments, he thought his analytic function was being preserved and believed that if he persevered in his work the symbolic network would be amplified. After the acute enactment he realized that he had not in fact been fully aware of his involvement in the dual collusions. Second, after the acute enactments, the analyst believed that he had lost his analytic capacity. Afterwards, he realized that he had in fact regained it. His impression of having traumatized his patient was replaced by surprise in finding that the analytic process was developing with dreams-for two. The dual collusion had been undone, which enabled access to the triangular reality.

There are times when the triangular reality imposes itself and the dyad fails to maintain this traumatic perception, so the dual collusion is remade. These situations must recur many times as ways of mourning are developed for the loss of the dual relationship and while the symbolic network is being repaired. The acute enactment is utilized when there is sufficient repair for the trauma to be tolerated and dreamed.

Broadening the understanding of chronic enactment, we can also assume that it freezes traumas inscribed in the unrepressed unconscious (Freud, 1923), which includes transgenerational events. The analytic field is taken over by archaic configurations dramatized by both members of the dyad, who may remain unaware of this. The dramatization can take different expressive forms manifested through actions, mimicry, emotions, sounds, smells, forms of language construction, tones, timbres of voice. They can take ideopicto- graphic forms like theatrical mime or silent cinema (Sapisochin, 2013). This expressivity can be very subtle in its visible manifestations, and very potent in its capacity for emotional involvement. When dealing with adolescent detachment we can take as models the various scenes drawn from the myths of Narcissus and Oedipus, for example.[8]

Theories and conjectures: Oedipus and Katia

This chapter has described the vicissitudes of adolescence, emphasizing the varying degrees of oscillation between dual and triangular relationships, keeping the reliving of oedipal situations as a framework. Now we shall address the complexity of these situations in comparing Oedipus and Katia. This involves condensed imaginative conjectures (Bion, 1970), dreams of vigil in which the vicissitudes of both adolescents are imagined. These conjectures refer to re-interpretations of aspects of the oedipal myth which can serve as a model for technical aspects.

Oedipus hears rumours (from inside and outside his mind) that he is an illegitimate child. Traumatized, he leaves Corinth in search of himself. He does not consciously know what he is doing but seeks to differentiate himself from his adoptive parents, who prevented him from coming into contact with reality. They had deceived him; he had not even been informed that he was adopted and was being prepared, as a prince, to maintain the symbiosis of the Royal Family. His first stop is the oracle of Delphi where he must spend the night dreaming. The priest will make his predictions from listening to him recount his dreams. He endures a terrible night haunted by scenes of terror which repeat themselves compulsively. He cannot tell whether they are nightmares or reality. He desperately tries to put them into words for the priest: the earth was quaking, mountains were crumbling, a seductive woman was crying? But, being a prince, as he speaks he seeks to maintain an air of arrogant indifference. After hearing his account, the priest accuses him of being a future criminal who will murder his father and marry his mother. The priest calls the guards and Oedipus is expelled from the temple. He hears the furious crowd clamouring for his death. Is this happening inside or outside his mind? Oedipus flees in despair on the brink of annihilation, and runs aimlessly, like a madman.

Adolescent Katia leaves her city and goes to H. She does not know it, but she is trying to escape from the family symbiosis, risking herself in search of herself. She is also fleeing the realization of the threat of the death of her oedipal rival. At her first stop, university, she suffers a terrible trauma. She was being persecuted and drugged (by rival colleagues or by the drug already within her?). She felt overwhelmed with confusion in the form of uncontrollable desires – competitive, murderous, envious, sexual (results of the internal drug ...). In truth, she would not even know what to call them. A crowd of colleagues and teachers (could they be parents and siblings?) wanted to either seduce her or kill her. Or is this what she herself wanted? She was confused as to whether these were real events, nightmares or hallucinations. Perhaps they were all these things at once. At other times she felt superior, she was directly connected to God, she was all-powerful. Sometimes she cried miserably, she missed being the little princess of the Royal Palace where she was looked after by her parents, the King and Queen, and by a battalion of servants who anticipated her desires even before she could. Who knows? If she died she might then be able to return to this paradise world (Cassorla, 1997b, 2000).

But hell compulsively returns. And Katia flees like a madwoman through the streets and down the highway of life.

As adolescents, Oedipus and Katia relive traumatic primitive situations. In the myth, Oedipus was branded with the terrible threat of death. He was undesirable, and at birth he did not find someone who could contain his terrors of annihilation. He was abandoned and left to die on Mount Cithaeron. These terrors are relived in the temple of Apollo, where he is condemned and abandoned by the priest. The priest behaves like a stupid analyst recruited by massive projective identifications. Oedipus does not understand his fate to be parricidal and incestuous. It is only after this discovery that he realizes why his parents wanted to kill him as a baby: the parricide was within him before he was born (along with the incestuous desire) and now that he is strong enough to kill (and his body to copulate) he feels more terrified. But nothing is clear to him.

Through her adolescent terrors, Katia relives traumas similar to those of the initial detachment. Traumatic signs of death are inscribed in her mind, of which transgenerational symbiotic defensive fusions form a component. Katia fails in her attempt to undo them and tries desperately to achieve symbiosis with friends and boyfriends. When they do not latch on to her and insist upon being non-self, Katia feels annihilated. She flees in panic, not knowing where to go, until she finds something or someone with whom she tries to merge. Her mother's illness contributes to these situations. When Katia finds the oracle, her former therapist, the latter calls her crazy. Desperate and terrified, Katia becomes even crazier.

Katia imagines she can escape from madness by merging with God, with her boyfriend, with drugs. Oedipus imagines he can escape from the madness that was projected onto him in Corinth. Fleeing far away will surely prevent him from killing his father or committing incest. But he is unable to flee far from his mind. I have the image of Oedipus despairing, walking down the road, hating himself and the world. He thinks it would be better to die. At a crossroads another obstacle presents itself: in the road ahead of him there is a cart and an arrogant, armed man. If Oedipus were dead, everything would be resolved. To bring about his own death would be a "homicide precipitated by the victim" (Cassorla, 1997b, 2000). The adolescent and the man argue over the way. But Oedipus's hatred and his desire for vengeance is greater than his desire to die. Oedipus kills the man. This man was Laius, his father, but he was unaware of this. Initially Oedipus feels better, but soon the melancholy guilt takes hold of him. This time the guilt is even greater, and Oedipus does not know why.

In her mind, Katia kills her rival mother. Her mother and the dead parental couple become mortiferous, so Katia is attacked from within. Guilty and destroyed, she has no one to turn to for help. She returns home and locks herself in her room, imagining that in this cloister of sorts she can hide from her crimes. Like Narcissus, she does not want to address any demands but the mirror and the Internet. She sleeps using narcotics (derived from *narcissus*) which cause nightmarish non-dreams. She gets involved in gossip on social networking sites where being noticed by others makes her feel like she exists (Levy, 2006). She despairs. She searches for a new oracle. That turns out to be me, her analyst. She presents me with riddles and then hides them from me. She wants and at the same time does not want to know who she is, who she was, who she will be. I investigate and set her new riddles. She flees, then she clings on, all at the same time.

Oedipus encounters the Sphinx, a kind of oracle who kills young people who fail to solve her riddles. His desire to die has returned, stronger this time. His morbid curiosity and his arrogant stupidity make the Sphinx seem increasingly attractive. He has nothing to lose – death would be welcome. Will his death bring him into symbiosis with the mother-Sphinx? The Sphinx terrorizes others because she is herself terrified. Looking at her, Oedipus is able to grasp this terror so similar to his own. He is sympathetic and tries to understand her as he is trying to understand himself. He has already come a long way down this road, and he has learnt a thing or two. He knows what it is to crawl on all fours on the stony ground; he knows from when he tried to walk with his two painful feet and had to use a stick. The stick becomes his third foot which will be replaced, in old age, by the support of his daughter, Antigone. He needs help to support his traumatized mind. Oedipus dreams these emotional experiences and solves the Riddle. Now he lives in the triangular reality and is able to think and dream. When Oedipus is no longer in need of the prosthetic mother-Sphinx she, like a good analyst, symbolically kills herself.

Katia also seeks the peace that she has lost in death. The drugs have the same effect. Katia searches for the Sphinx-analyst who can help her think through her riddles. With much back and forth, this process continues.

Oedipus marries Jocasta, they have children, and his reign is a happy one. That is, until the arrival of the plague. This internal plague is the reliving of the incestuous and homicidal impulses which emerge when Oedipus reaches the same age his father Laius had been when he was killed. His eldest son also happens to be the same age that Oedipus had been when he killed Laius. The identification configurations are activated like Anniversary Reactions (Cassorla 1986, 1991b, 2008b). As a pseudomature adolescent, Oedipus experiences a psychotic break in mature age (Ungar, 2004).

The oracle predicts that the plague (madness) will cease when Laius's murderer is discovered. This is where Sophocles begins *Oedipus Rex* and the tragedy of us all, which in truth has no beginning. It is an eternal return.

Conclusions

Working with adolescents requires the analyst's constant attention in identifying situations into which he could be drawn by defences that form a part of the detachment process. Numbed perception normally threatens when the analyst confuses himself with the concomitance of dual and triangular relationships, or as a result of the speed of the oscillations between the two. These threats are usually rapidly undone, thanks to the analytic function.

However, when the young patient and their family organize stable defensive conglomerates the analyst runs the risk of allowing himself to be drawn in to such a degree that he becomes stupid. The analyst must be wary of situations in which the analytic process seems to be proceeding "very well". It is possible that he is being drawn into mutually idealized collusions with the young patient and their family. On the other hand, the analyst who has difficulties in perceiving his own fear or anger may be vulnerable to blackmail and threats from the young patient and their family without fully realizing it. These situations occur when the projective identifications become entangled with the professional's personal conflicts.

Sessions with the family are a necessary component of working with young people, as much to undo mutual fantasies as to understand what is going on. Referral to other analysts may be necessary. Symbiotic families may prematurely remove the young person from analysis if this symbiosis is not addressed. The analyst, in particular the more inexperienced, can be subtly recruited to take the side of the parents and of society against the adolescent. The contrary may also occur: the analyst identifies with the rebellious or inquisitive adolescent who can feel like a victim of adults. These situations stem from the analyst's insufficiently developed conflicts in relation to his own adolescence. These conflicts are made possible by the projective identifications of the young person, the parents, and other people around them.

I hope that the models discussed in this text will help the analysts of adolescents to identify such signals early, and undo situations in which there is the risk of pathological involvement with defensive organizations, all the while bearing in mind the environment and society in which the adolescent lives.

Notes

1 This chapter was originally published as Stupidity in the analytic field: vicissitudes of the detachment process in adolescence. In: *The International Journal of Psychoanalysis* 98(2): 371–391 (2017). DOI: 10.1111/1745–8315.12577, copyright © Institute of Psychoanalysis, reprinted by permission of Taylor & Francis Ltd, www.tandfonline.com on behalf of Institute of Psychoanalysis.

2 Tiresias latches onto Oedipus's dilemmas, which mobilizes his own 'oedipal' conflicts. These are mythically exposed in his interference with the Zeus–Hera couple and in his killing of snakes engaged in the sexual act (Cassorla, 2008b, 2010b).

3 The construction of clinical material conforms to standards of confidentiality as recommended by Gabbard (2000).

4 The "turning a blind eye" mechanism was described by Steiner (1985); it is applied by Cassorla (1993) in the clinic in cases of emotional blindness.
5 The patient is expelled from Paradise and thrown into Hell. If this Hell could be dreamed it would be transformed into Earth and into reality. But the demons of Hell and the idealized gods will always continue to haunt the patient (Cassorla, 2010a).
6 A review of these authors' ideas can be found in Cassorla (1997a, 2004, 2008c) and Brown (2011). This author studies the question of intersubjectivity in great depth. The evolution of the concept of Projective Identification may be found in Spillius & O'Shaughnessy (2011).
7 The development of ideas regarding chronic and acute enactments can be found in Cassorla (2001, 2005, 2008a, 2012, 2014).
8 The ideas about enactment were developed after the publication of this paper in R. M.S. Cassorla (2018). *The Psychoanalyst, the Theatre of Dreams and the Clinic of Enactment*. London: Routledge.

References

Aberastury, A. (1980). *Adolescência*. Porto Alegre: Artes Médicas.

Baranger, M. & Baranger, W. (1968[1961–62]). The analytic situation as a dynamic field. *International Journal of Psychoanalysis* 89: 795–826.

Baranger, M., Baranger, W. & Mom, J. (1983). Process and non-process in analytic work. *International Journal of Psychoanalysis* 64: 1–15.

Barros, E.M.R. (2011). Reflections on the clinical implication of symbolism. *International Journal of Psychoanalysis* 92: 879–901.

Bion, W.R. (1961). *Experiences in Groups*. London: Routledge.

Bion, W.R. (1962). *Learning from Experience*. London: Heinemann.

Bion, W.R. (1967). On Arrogance. In: *Second Thoughts – Selected Papers on Psycho-Analysis*. London: Heinemann, pp. 86–92.

Bion, W.R. (1970). *Attention and Interpretation*. London: Tavistock Publications.

Bleger, J. (1967). *Simbiosis y ambigüedad*. Buenos Aires: Paidós.

Blos, P. (1962). *On Adolescence: A Psychoanalytic Interpretation*. Glencoe, IL: Free Press.

Bolognini, S. (2004). O bar no deserto. Simetria e assimetria no tratamento de adolescents difíceis. *Revista Brasileira de Psicanálise* 38(2): 259–269.

Brown, L.J. (2011). *Intersubjective Processes and the Unconscious: An Integration of Freudian, Kleinian and Bionian Perspectives*. New York: Routledge.

Casssorla, R.M.S. (1985). Depression and suicide in adolescence. In: Pan American Health Association (ed.). *The Health of Adolescents and Youths in the Americas*. Washington: PAHO, pp. 156–169.

Casssorla, R.M.S. (1986). Reações de aniversário: aspectos clínicos e teóricos. *Jornal de Psicanálise (São Paulo)* 19(38): 25–39.

Casssorla, R.M.S. (1991a). Simbiose na adolescência: implicações clínicas. In:Maakaroun, M., Souza, R.P. & Cruz, A.R. (eds), *Tratado de adolescência: um estudo multi-disciplinar*. Rio de Janeiro: Cultura Médica, pp. 514–523.

Casssorla, R.M.S. (1991b). O tempo a morte e as reações de aniversário. In:Cassorla, R.M.S. (Org). *Do suicídio: estudos brasileiros*. Campinas: Papirus, pp. 61–88.

Casssorla, R.M.S. (1993). Complexo de Édipo, curiosidade, vista grossa e catástrofe psicológica. *Revista Brasileira de Psicanálise* 27(4): 607–626.

Casssorla, R.M.S. (1997a). No emaranhado de identificações projetivas cruzadas com adolescentes e seus pais. *Revista Brasileira de Psicanálise* 31(3): 639–676.

Casssorla, R.M.S. (1997b). Comportamento suicida na adolescência: aspectos psi-cossociais. In: Levisky, D.L. (Org). *Adolescência e violência: consequências da realidade brasileira*. Porto Alegre:Artes Médicas, pp. 81–98.

Casssorla, R.M.S. (2000). Reflexões sobre teoria e técnica com pacientes potencialmente suicidas. *Alter – Jornal de Estudos Psicodinâmicos (Brasilia)* Pt 1, 19(2): 169–186; Pt 2, 19(2): 367–386.

Casssorla, R.M.S. (2001). Acute enactment as resource in disclosing a collusion between the analytical dyad. *International Journal of Psychoanalysis* 82(6): 1155–1170.

Casssorla, R.M.S.. (2004). In der Verwicklung von projectiven Kreuzidentifizierungen mit Adoleszenten und ihren Eltern. *Kinderanalyse* (Stuttgart) 3(12): 183–230.

Casssorla, R.M.S. (2005). From bastion to enactment: The 'non-dream' in the theatre of analysis. *International Journal of Psychoanalysis* 86(3): 699–719.

Casssorla, R.M.S. (2008a). The analyst's implicit alpha-function, trauma and enactment in the analysis of borderline patients. *International Journal of Psychoanalisis* 89(1): 161–180.

Casssorla, R.M.S. (2008b). Desvelando configurações emocionais da dupla analítica através de modelos inspirados no mito edípico. *Revista Brasileira de Psicoterapia (Porto Alegre)* 10: 37–48.

Casssorla, R.M.S. (2008c). O analista, seu paciente e a psicanálise contemporânea: considerações sobre indução mútua, enactment e não-sonho-a-dois. *Revista Latinoamericana de Psicoanálisis* 8: 189–208.

Casssorla, R.M.S. (2009). O analista, seu paciente adolescente e a psicanálise atual: sete reflexões. *Revista de Psicanálise de Porto Alegre)* 16(2): 261–278.

Casssorla, R.M.S. (2010a). A leste do Éden: loucura, feitiço e suicídio. *Revista Brasileira de Psicanálise* 44(2): 147–157.

Casssorla, R.M.S. (2010b). Édipo, Tirésias, o oráculo e a esfinge: do não-sonho às transformações em sonho. In: Rezze, C.J., Marra, E.S. & Petricciani, M. (Org). *Psicanálise: Bion. Teoria e Clínica*. São Paulo: Vetor, pp. 110–131.

Casssorla, R.M.S. (2012). What happens before and after acute enactment? An exercise in clinical validation and broadening of hypothesis. *International Journal of Psychoanalysis* 93(1): 53–89.

Casssorla, R.M.S. (2013a). Reflections on Non-dreams-for-two, Enactment and the Analyst's Implicit Alpha-function. In:Levine, H.B. & Brown, L.J., *Growth and Turbulence in the Container/Contained: Bion's Continuing Legacy*. New York: Routledge, pp. 151–176.

Casssorla, R.M.S. (2013b). In search of symbolization. The analyst task of dreaming. In: Levine, H., Reed, G. & Scarfone, D. (eds). *Unrepresented States and the Construction of Meaning. Clinical and Theoretical Contributions*. London: Karnac Books, pp. 202–219.

Casssorla, R.M.S. (2013c). When the analyst becomes stupid: an attempt to understand enactment using Bion's theory of thinking. *Psychoanalytic Quarterly* 82(2): 323–360.

Casssorla, R.M.S. (2014). The silent movie: discussion of the case Ellen. *International Journal of Psychoanalysis* 95: 93–102.

Cassorla, R.M.S. (2018). *The Psychoanalyst, the Theatre of Dreams and the Clinic of Enactment*. London: Routledge.

Faimberg, H. (1996). Listening to listening. *International Journal of Psychoanalysis* 77(4): 667–677.

Freud, S. (1893). Studies on Hysteria (Case Histories). *S.E.* II. London: Hogarth Press.

Freud, S. (1905). Fragment of an Analysis of a Case of Hysteria. *S.E.* VII. London: The Hogarth Press.

Freud, S. (1923). The Ego and the Id. *S.E.* XIX. London: The Hogarth Press.

Gabbard, G.O. (2000). Disguise or consent: problems and recommendations concerning the publication and presentation of clinical material. *International Journal of Psychoanalysis* 81(6): 1071–1086.

Grinberg, L. (1976). *Teoria de la identificación.* Buenos Aires: Paidós.

Joseph, B. (1989). *Psychic Equilibrium and Psychic Change: Selected Papers of Betty Joseph,* ed. Feldman, M. & Spillius, E.B.London: Routledge.

Levy, R. (1996). Refúgios narcisistas na adolescência: entre a busca de proteção e o risco de destruição-dilemas na contratransferência. *Revista Brasileira de Psicanálise* 30(1): 223–240.

Levy, R. (2006). Adolescência: o reordenamento simbólico, o olhar e o equilíbrio narcísico. *Revista de Psicanálise (Porto Alegre)* 13(2): 233–245.

Mahler, M. (1968). *On Human Symbiosis and the Vicissitudes of Individuation.* New York: International Universities Press.

Meltzer, D. (1966). The relation of anal masturbation to projective identification. *International Journal of Psychoanalysis* 47(2): 335–343.

Meltzer, D. (1973). *Sexual States of Mind.* Perthshire: Clunie Press.

Meltzer, D. (1992). *The Claustrum: An Investigation of Claustrophobic Phenomena.* Perthshire: Clunie Press.

Paz, L.R. (1980) *Adolescência – crise de dessimbiotização.* In: Aberastury, A., *Adolescência.* Porto Alegre: Artes Médicas, pp. 165–184.

Rosenfeld, H. (1987). *Impasse and Interpretation.* London: Tavistock Publications.

Sapisochin, S. (2013). Second thoughts on Agieren: listening the enacted. *International Journal of Psychoanalysis* 94(5): 967–991.

Spillius, E.B. & O' Shaughnessy, E. (eds) (2012). *Projective Identification: The Fate of a Concept.* New York: Routledge.

Steiner, J. (1985). Turning a blind-eye: the cover up for Oedipus. *International Review of Psycho-Analysis* 12(2): 161–172.

Steiner, J. (1993). *Psychic Retreats: Pathological Organizations in Psychotic, Neurotic and Borderline Patients.* London: Routledge.

Ungar, V. (2004). O trabalho psicanalítico com adolescentes, hoje. *Revista Brasileira de Psicanálise* 38(3): 735–749.

Ungar, V. (2013). La fin de l'adolescence aujourd'hui. *Revue française de psychanalyse* 77(2): 376–391.

Winnicott, D. (1949). Hate in the countertransference. *International Journal of Psychoanalysis* 30: 69–75.

2 Cherchez la femme – becoming a woman

The mother-daughter relationship during adolescence

Silvia Flechner

Preliminary considerations

The feminine and maternal world is considered a field marked with events of enormous unrest and high intensity, generating deep marks and unfathomable traumas repeated transgenerationally, over the centuries, being maintained even in our current times.

History and religions have been eloquent regarding women. Let us take the Council of Trent (1545) as an example. It was during that Council that Catholicism recognized that women had a soul. Likewise, since the end of the 18th century, during the French Revolution (1789), women's rights began to be asserted; however, the leaders of this revolution argued that freedom, equality, and fraternity only applied to men. Later, Napoleon would subject women to even stricter male authority through legislative code.

Throughout history, in all civilizations, the myth of matriarchy has not reflected a historical reality of female dominance, but a very different anthropological reality. Being born a woman concedes the possibility of being a mother. Many women are mothers because they want to, others because it is an obligation. Some mothers love or always claim to love their children. Others claim that sometimes they love them and sometimes they do not. Other mothers do not love their children, do not say they love them, and do not demonstrate it with their actions. There are controlling, invasive, aggressive, violent, homicidal, phallic, castrating, incestuous, affectionate, loved, and hated mothers, as many as there have been mothers throughout time. Some mothers have never wanted to be mothers and there are women who did want to be mothers, but science was not yet sufficiently prepared for them to be mothers.

The current 21st-century society in which we live makes it clear that many women do not want to have children; the birth rate in Western countries is worryingly decreasing for those for whom this fact has become a problem due to different interests. On the other hand, we now have advanced scientific means to allow women who want to be mothers to do so through increasingly sophisticated processes. The freezing of eggs, in vitro fertilization, egg donation, and storage of sperm or eggs before cancer treatment in children and

DOI: 10.4324/9781003380283-2

adolescents are all options. In addition, transgender couples and surrogates have desires for a child. These are some of the circumstances that force us to reconsider the clinic we are facing today. Is it perhaps the power of science and genetics that is getting the upper hand on what was considered the act of intercourse of a "couple"?

What does the birth of another human being mean for each mother-to-be? A magical moment, an endless effort, a feeling of emotion as old as humanity, an absolute rejection of the newborn, as many feelings, affections, and sensations as there have been mothers in the world.

Despite all the efforts observed in many women to radically cut their ties with family traditions, a pregnancy will forcefully resurface fantasies regarding their mother. The mother who was a daughter a short time ago will now have to repeat the action of bringing a baby into the world.

Unresolved conflicts with the maternal image will inevitably influence the repetition of the procreative act; this will have been systematically expelled from consciousness and repressed. Each mother has also been a daughter; therefore, she brings a transgenerational history that will be repeated in some way, as Faimberg (2005) has pointed out in the telescoping of generations. It also happens with the father, or his substitute, loved or hated, often reliving a poorly resolved Oedipus.

The birth of a child will generate a primary link with the mother that will intertwine between the psychic and the corporal, building a common kind of cover for both before progressively differentiating perception and object representation. The baby will become, for a while (if all goes well), her choice of erotic object. According to the relationship type and the separation form between mother and daughter, a complex, singular, and unique relationship will emerge. Separation anxieties play an essential role since it is anxiety about a loss of union that is irremediable. Separation, on the other hand, allows the beginning of the making up of her own story in the new psychosexual framework of the girl.

Female sexuality, the mother-daughter conflict

Anna O., Dora, and Caterina are some names of the famous cases that were the paradigmatic women in Freud's first discoveries. Hysteria was imposed as the "model of all psychoneuroses" because they combine "a sexual repression that exceeds dimension" and "an excessive development of the sexual drive," as explained by Freud (1923).

However, André (1994) points out that, according to Freud, masculine sexuality will never be the object of isolated treatment. In Freud's mind, only femininity required a boundary. Starting from the idea of a common androcentric core, as if the libido itself --- the energy of the sexual drive – was virile or masculine, he thus placed the accent on female sexuality. The rupture is fierce between the Oedipal story of the girl (typically related to her father) and the prehistory of the complex (which is tied between mother and daughter), it is very different from the continuity that characterizes the psychosexual development of the male.

Freud particularly stresses the ambivalence of this first union, the hostility of which the mother is the object as strongly as the love directed towards her. Why such a marked ambivalence? To answer this question, André suggests that it will be necessary to consider the intersubjective point of view. Let us note that the maternal and paternal unconscious is mainly absent from these Freudian texts on femininity. The first instances of sexual life are also marked by the unconscious relationship of the mother to the daughter and of the daughter to the mother; what happens with and in the daughter will be inextricable from the maternal unconscious representations.

To be able to face one's own story, the psychic work to be carried out will be intense, with its rhythm exploring the limits, often going beyond them. The result of differentiation that is put into play in the daughter ought to offer her the possibility of affirming the differences established between her and her mother. For this, it will be necessary to eradicate the narcissistic cover that attracted them and that they shared earlier.

Chabert (2013) accounts for the consubstantiality between anxieties and separation, stating that castration anguish, loss of love by the object anguish, and annihilation anguish each refer to a separation work. Regardless of its form, the attempt will be to separate either from the illusory omnipotent belief, from the first objects of love, from oneself and life when we speak of annihilation anxieties.

Thinking about the work throughout life, we notice that what had been conferred as essential has ceased to be so; therefore, all changes imply a separation from who, at another time, was there and who, at some point, we will have to resign.

Between love and hate, identification and rejection, the relationship between mother and daughter in adolescence is full of conflict. The identifications can oscillate from a specular coincidence until reaching the resounding rejection, with different degrees of intensity between said identifications. The cohesion of the beginnings should usually be weakened; the assumption of rejection and hatred towards the mother by the adolescent will allow her to trace her subjectivation paths. If this path is achieved, the young girls will take their peer group as the closest reference since they are in a comparable situation.

The position of union-separation is where different states and affections are put into play, such as anguish, fascination, ambivalence, and guilt, until it is replaced by symbolic death that implies ending the mourning for the loss of childhood and child parents, as well as ceasing to be "the wonderful girl" of those parents.

Through transformation and modification work, adolescents manage to appropriate themselves, even though, on many occasions, the road is extremely rocky. Nevertheless, this appropriation reveals the inner feminine that is simultaneously imperceptible and disturbing, thus producing a fragile and constant balance-imbalance, unsustainable, that shows the difficulty of developing a filiation trapped between a relationship marked by excesses and rupture.

The suffering of the adolescent during this elaboration impasse can lead to existential pain that can be staged in different ways, be it attacks against one's own body, depressive or melancholic symptoms, eating disorders, addictions, etc. These psychopathological manifestations will cover the oedipal conflict that may be disfigured or deformed. Moreover, these psychopathological states can account for an unavoidable absence by the mother and a complicated environment.

It will be necessary for the analyst to consider dangerous situations such as deadly regression or risk of counterphobia that manage to leave the path open to hazardous actions. Extremely narcissistic mothers who fail to vest their daughters can generate considerably harmful situations for adolescents.

For example, in my work with anorexic patients, I have made enormous progress in patient recovery. At the same time, a patient's mother, "in a moment of distraction", telephoned me in anguish because she had "inadvertently" gave her daughter one of her slimming tablets.

Both anorexia and bulimia reveal a failure to elaborate specifically on feminine anxieties. Throughout a woman's life, both what enters the female body (food, sexual relations, etc.) and what comes out (menstrual blood) requires work of elaboration on what femininity implies.

An undifferentiated adolescent body – usually female – can express internal and external conflicts, where the symptoms related to eating disorders occupy a privileged place. The pubertal irruption can overflow the continence capacity of a psychic space that until then was governed by infantile sexuality and by the fantasized image of idealized parents.

The most to be expected of her will be demonstrated by the fact that the adolescent manages to discover the woman in herself – if that is her desire – detaching herself from the internal image of the intrusive and violent mother, preserving the hope that the mother has the capacity to accompany somehow this problematic passage of his daughter.

Working with adolescents is the privileged ground in dealing with life, sexuality, acting, confrontation, and death. The drive movements are played peculiarly, primarily reflected through performances or passages to acts. Acting that, in many cases, takes the shape of an intrusive and violent act for the adolescent himself or their environment that can often end with death.

The maternal function

Winnicott (1990) has highlighted the role of the mother in providing the baby with the elements of reality with which to build a psychic image of the external world. The mother's role as an auxiliary self in the beginning, through holding, handling, and presenting objects, allows the baby to live and grow under the illusion of primary omnipotence.

The maternal function cannot be dissociated from the feminine enigma. Wishing to have a child, on the one hand, implies thinking of oneself as desiring. On the other, it is thinking of oneself with the ambivalence a woman experiences during pregnancy, of the baby's birth.

The newborn is, above all, a fragile being, a disorganized set of impulses and perceptions that demonstrate the absolute dependence and the need for that auxiliary self (usually the mother) that allows to integrate bodily sensations, environmental stimuli, and emerging motor skills.

The enigma arises at each birth concerning the maternal emotional situation. When the mother cannot provide the necessary protection and support to the newborn, there will be a perception on the part of the newborn of a lack, perceiving the environment as threatening.

The personality construction and maternal psychopathology can place the psychic structure of the newborn at high risk. In addition, depressions, mistreatment due to depression, absences, and risk situations always lead us to investigate the family history of the mother as well as concerns of symbiotic unions and fusional states that also appear and may be based on the maternal family history.

The clinic shows us that at a certain point, women leave a man's field of desire to narcissistically hold on to an eternal return to their mother, an omnipotent mother whom they cannot abandon. That desired and hated mother is the maternal object that will remain as an infinite identity reference, and she will then leave an indelible trace. Thus, their love relationships will have the character of a partial object and not become a different genital object.

This situation refers to the image of a hypothetical original union, an archaic relationship that excludes the father or any third party where, according to McDougall (1966), there will be an absence in the difference between love and hate, which in turn results in a denial of time and history, suppressing all possible tension and change.

A stranger to herself, the young woman may begin to show self-harming behaviours, a drastic control, impossible to enact over her own body that will lead her to a confinement that will bring about the effect of desire for non-desire. Faced with such excess or invasion, an enigmatic form of anguish arises which, according to Aulagnier (2003), could be read as "the energy in action in the psychic space, which is responsible for what we define as the desire of a non-desire: a desire not to have to desire, such is the other characteristic object of all desire." Such a desire, that is, to not have desire (for example, in the case of self-harm) would be arranged as a desire not to live life but to endure it, an ambiguous limit to which the ego is a hostage.

We cannot ignore that, on many occasions, mother and daughter will be in the same era of femininity. Especially in current times, where the ideal of youth is highly valued, jealousy and envy of the young and seductive female body are often a source of conflict. It was a fairly common situation for the daughter to search among the mother's clothes for the first garments to start a path toward femininity. Instead, today we see reverse conditions, it is now the mother who wishes to wear her daughter's clothes, reflecting a desire for eternal youth.

Francesca: Actions speak louder than words

For years I have worked with adolescents at serious risk; many of these situations have touched me and resulted in the fundamental understanding that it is necessary to give the adolescent space and time during the adolescent transition that sometimes differs from the usual ways in which we work. The risk situations to which the adolescent is exposed can come from the interior world due to the transformation of psychic changes and the sexually mature body. They may also involve family circumstances, exposing the adolescent to traumatic situations that are sometimes irreparable. The adolescent's situation, as well as the family nucleus, can lead to extreme family events that acting and acting out can emerge before the beginning of psychoanalytic treatment and throughout it.

Francesca was 17 years old; she was a very thin young woman when she came to see me after the death of her mother who had committed suicide by jumping from her 14th-floor apartment. Her mother had suffered from severe depression for many years. Much later in her analysis, I captured a variety of maternal psychotic disorders, which were also present in her behaviour. It was clear that her mother had not been treated appropriately, nor was she hospitalized despite specific warnings that reported the possibility of suicide.

Francesca was the only family member in her home on the day of her death. Her mother asked her daughter for some pants since she had lost weight. "It's until I gain weight." Those were practically her last words to Francesca. She then locked herself in the bathroom with a window overlooking an air shaft. Noticing that her mother had remained there for too long, Francesca knocked on the bathroom door. She insisted, called her, and yelled for her to get out. She suddenly heard her mother cry, but even so, her mother did not answer her. She called her father, who arrived immediately, having been warned for a long time of the seriousness of his wife's condition. Despite her father's intense screams, she did not open the door either; therefore, he forced and pushed it down. When he succeeded, they saw the mother's feet falling into the void. Francesca went into shock.

The beginning of the treatment was challenging; between remembering and not wanting to do it, added to not wanting to speak, between crying, sorrow, and anger, Francesca found herself unable, above all, to express guilt on the one hand and on the other the anger she felt towards her mother. It was difficult for her to find the words that would betray her anger. This anger has accompanied her for many years now. The feeling of abandonment by her mother towards her had started very early in her life.

As a child, she had suffered bullying at school but never dared to report it; she could not share practically any activity with her mother because she was always tired, lying down, waiting for her husband to arrive to take care of their daughter and home. Francesca noticed that her father had much character, he was a hard-working man, not very affectionate, but she also saw that her mother dominated him.

After the treatment was consolidated, her transference-countertransference axis slowly strengthened until she began to talk about her mother. Thus, she could recount what Francesca called "the assassination attempts of her mother or not wanting to die alone."

A year ago, her mother had been driving, accompanied by her daughter, and suddenly she began to accelerate in such a way that Francesca asked her to slow down, When she did not receive, she began to yell at her and told her that she was going to open the car door even with the car in motion. Finally, her mother stopped the car, and Francesca warned her: "If you want to kill yourself, do it alone," adding that she should not kill her, thus getting out of her car. Several similar situations were revealed over more than a decade of analysis.

Faced with this valuable remembrance of this terrible memory, Francesca could recognize that a part of her knew that her mother was at serious risk. She was also able to associate it with the fact that her suicide was carried out while wearing her daughter's pants.

A part of Francesca died with her mother – symbolized not only by her pants – without yet being able to elaborate on such mourning. Nevertheless, numerous marks were left on Francesca after her mother's death; these were later represented in acts whose repetition clearly showed the force of the death drive. Although it was not the only one, one related to opening the car door while it was moving and her father was driving.

Staying with Freud, let us consider the changes he later included in "Beyond the Pleasure Principle" (Freud, 1920). The death drive will give the repetition compulsion a new meta-psychological status. Something likely to be repeated through acting (Agieren) not only concerns the repressed or the hallucinatory satisfaction of desire, except for extrapolating the set of potentially traumatic experiences, but also has not accessed a representation, nor has it been integrated into the psyche.

Whatever the objective of the psychoanalytic situation is then the fundamental zone of the unconscious drive, that intractable zone that resists the treatment of representation and memory, what the analyst renounces and forces to regulate the listening, on what the patient does not know that he knows, and the analyst cannot go further.

The failures in the foundations of the development of the ego and its consequent repercussion in the access to the symbolic or in the relationship with the other lead us to think about a situation of fusion between one's own and the other. The ego may be driven to act out a tragic scene due to the lack of symbolic mediations, hardly accessing sadomasochistic representations, perhaps because, in adolescence, the ego finds itself overwhelmed by the demands of the drive and its context.

As the analysis progressed, I noticed difficulties in Francesca that stemmed from a malfunction between mother and daughter and within the family environment. What could not be verbalized appeared in scenes that took place outside of the session. The unexpected and traumatic death of the mother resulted in a state of false maturity in needing to care for her disturbed father. Simultaneously, she was permanently in the shadow of the traumatic memory in an unthinkable way.

Still, unrepresentable violence also disturbed the process of analysis and her capacity for symbolization. This violence was observed in how she entered the office, with a kind of arrogance or pride that thus prevented any approach, even in greeting. After a few minutes of starting the session, she seemed to have only just arrived. The defensive mechanisms that placed her on high alert could not allow her to approach the other, and also did prevent her talking to anyone other than her analyst. Her friends had been rejected, and she remained convinced in the belief that her father could not comfort her because he was the one who needed her help.

As I was arranged as a reference point by her, I tried, again and again, to understand why she was convinced that her father could neither comfort nor protect her. She finally stood up and yelled at me, "You don't understand anything! A man locked in his room, and when you open the door, he has a thousand photos of my mother stuck to all the walls, can't help me!"

I then realized that my role as an analyst – at least for a while – would have to be as support on a much larger scale than the way in which I had been used to working.

We cannot evoke the traumatic transgenerational aspect of family history without thinking of a melancholic nucleus that is also transmitted. It will be the shadow of the traumatic event where memory has sometimes been lost, or denied or split due to the effect of certain narcissistic pacts. (Kristeva, 1987). Godfrind (2018) joins Cournut-Janin's (1998) findings with respect to the melancholic core and notes the presence of a bewitching maternal imago with respect to the daughter, a link called *"primary homosexuality"*.

This traumatic situation evokes the impossibility of mourning, not being able to – in this case, the father – protect his daughter. Risk behaviours in Francesca increased with self-destructive attitudes, exposing a deadly, risky bias that remained floating in each session.

Specific dangerous ties between mother and daughter can disturb both the internal space and the external world. Becoming a woman exceeds the maternal and requires a particularly complex operation. This operation includes the various identification movements which Laplanche (1988) has called "enigmatic messages".

This is what Kahn (2018) refers to, stating that what is objective of the psychoanalytic situation is then the irreducible zone of the unconscious drive, that intractable zone that resists the treatment of representation and memory, what the analyst renounces and forces to regulate the listening, what the patient does not know that knows and the analyst cannot go further.

The importance that has been given to penis envy

The notion of penis envy, from the psychoanalytic point of view, has provoked numerous debates and polemics. We might think that the problem is not centred on the existence or not of such envy but rather on what place should be given to penis envy in the girl's psychosexual evolution?

Freud (1905) describes the triggering of penis envy in the girl remarking that "the penis, surprisingly visible and well-sized, of a brother or some playmate, immediately recognizes the superior counterpart of its own small and hidden organ and from then she succumbs to penis envy". Victim, "seriously" wounded, remains prey to a feeling of inferiority that will settle in the girl and then in the woman when she recognizes her "narcissistic wound". Thus, the girl sees what she does not have, this fact which leads to the enigma of the difference between sexes.

Among the representations caused by penis envy, André suggests one in particular: the castrating woman. His contribution, respect to the masculine unconscious is linked to the castration anxiety, favouring the construction of the character of the castrating woman.

During the castration complex of the male, the boy discovers that the female anatomy is different – women do not have a penis – assuming that they have been stripped of it, associating this fact with fantasized threats that the absence is due to castration. Subsequently, the boy will discover that his mother is a woman, and she does not possess it either; thus, the unconscious castration anxiety develops.

Volnovich (2010) mentions peculiarly that feared and hated for being castrated, the woman becomes the object of endless complaints about what we would like her to be or do and, she neither is nor does, the boring ones, the ones who daze us with their chatter, the fools who do not know how to earn a living. He also mentions it concerning the masculine discourse about fear and hatred of the castrating woman: Feared and hated for being "castrating," women receive complaints and blame for what we (men) are not. The woman criticizes our failures and is responsible for our limitations. These are the mothers who disempower us in front of our children, hypercritical of our weaknesses, "frigid," overwhelm us with their sexual claims, and treat us like we were children.

Volnovich affirms that heterosexual men have been trained to have sexual relations without paying the high price of the commitment of affective relationships, which are synonymous with an unacceptable weakness for those who wear the trousers well. "But there is a point at which patriarchal logic traps us: since men have often thought of women as their exclusive private property, the unhappiness and depression of our partners involve us more than necessary."

Freudian theory is typical of its time. Therefore, phallocentrism is found as one of its bases. Despite this, we know that the discovery of the unconscious and its theories on sexuality, among other topics, have become unquestionable as one of the most important revelations regarding the human being. However, some of its basic statements produce some discomfort regarding femininity: In *Three Essays on the Theory of Sexuality* (1905) Freud assumes that there is no primacy of the genitals – penis – but rather a primacy of the phallus: "Things cannot happen in the same way as in the male. For this reason, the feminist demand for equality between the sexes is not very valid here: the morphological difference requirement be externalized in diversities of psychic development." To paraphrase Napoleon, "anatomy is destiny."

According to Freud (1930), the Superego will be deficient in women; this has also been one of the most contentious issues in Freudian theory regarding his vision of women that is, his approach to the female Superego, and the hostility of women towards culture. To hypothesize, Freud suggests that the girl accepts castration as an accomplished fact, while the boy fears the possibility of consummation. For this reason, he excludes castration anxiety in the girl since she lacks a powerful motive to establish the superego.

Although the woman has actively participated in the French Revolution, her recognition has always been late. Currently, even the strength of feminism does not seem to be able to clarify the question of being a woman. It will be challenging to answer, especially in certain feminist groups, if the path to reaffirming a sexual identity is experienced as an assault upon the other sex.

The body: puberty and adolescence – genitality

The body will mark, in both sexes, the period of change from puberty to adolescence; however, we know that the psyche does not progress with these changes with the physiological speed of the body. Therefore, it could sometimes become threatening. The disturbing strangeness of the pubescent body will cause uncontrollable sensations of overwhelming transitions, impossible to manage.

The pubescent body turns out to be – just like the psyche – a body in transit, in a state of transformation in which psychic nature factors are involved from the beginning of life, as well as social and cultural ones. It implies ceasing to maintain the protective barrier from the external gaze, exposing in some way, internal emotions. For example, blushing becomes a characteristic manifestation of puberty and often appears with it, betraying the young woman and revealing in a certain way, her inner world.

The coexistence of two forms of the Oedipus complex, positive and negative, determines dialectic identifications that lead to loving or hating one of the parents and later, loving or hating the other. Both sexual objects can specifically mobilize different drive movements, which can be more libidinal or aggressive. The dynamics of fantasies are built on pairs of opposites: activity-passivity, masculine-feminine, sadism-masochism, and above all love and hate, allocating them to the father or mother.

The adolescent's ability is, among others, to transform (give a new form) what has been found until then in autoeroticism as destiny. The access to the genital sexual revolves and assumes the entrance to the oedipal problem. What is not genitalized during adolescence can embody the sign of difficulties about narcissistic conflicts during the movement from infantile to genital sexuality and adult sexuality.

However, adolescent, and adult sexuality is not reduced to genital; the genital sexual remains as a reference, as an organizer of human sexuality. We could say that genitality is based on infantile sexuality, as well as archaic sexuality, therefore accessing the continuity and growth of the subjective construction.

Child sexual life shows specific components that include – from the beginning – other subjects as sexual objects. From this perspective, it is to be noted that there might be partial drives, like pleasure in seeing or exhibiting cruelty, which appear in an independent form regarding the erogenous zones and would later come into action with genital life. The drive to see can emerge in the child as a spontaneous sexual expression developing a lively interest in the genitals of playmates.

Boys and girls also develop the cruel components of the sexual drive. Children characterized by particular cruelty towards animals and playmates could stir up suspicions of a premature and intense sexual practice coming from the erogenous zones. It is suggested that painful skin stimulation can be an erogenous stimulus.

But what happens when the reality is different, and we find ourselves working with adolescents on the edge? Because borderline states are today a consistent subjectivation model in adolescence. The difficulty seems to be focused on failed oedipal situations, the sociocultural crisis in which we are included, and the lack of internal possibilities that make it impossible to form a mature enough ego to face the current fragility of relations.

Homosexual relationships, often fleeting, among young people have become much more common than we suppose. It seems to have the nature of discovering sexes and could also be classified as a form of confrontation with maternal and paternal figures. Homosexual temptation in adolescence constitutes – among others – one of the ways of rejecting particular challenges to genitalization, especially the encounter with the other sex and reactivation of castration anxiety. It could be an economic solution, avoiding the confrontation with castration anxiety and anguish at the time in which the imminence of the encounter with the other sex is announced.

Bisexuality and neutral gender

Bisexuality, a concept introduced by Wilhelm Fliess in 1896, became a central notion in Freud's conceptualizations, that is, bisexuality is innate; the child is "originally" bisexual. Since his correspondence with Fliess, Freud had stressed the importance of bisexuality. The perverse-polymorphic disposition is common to all human beings, which allows them to put into practice all possible transgressions. Regardless of any identification or choice of object, subjectively, our sexuality is bisexual. In the same way as sexuality, bisexuality will conflict with necessary injunctions.

In a letter to Fliess, Freud (1896) used the word bisexuality for the first time. He said that to consider why the consequence of premature sexual experience is sometimes perversion and sometimes neurosis, "I benefit from the bisexuality of all human beings" (This also appears in "Analysis Terminable and Interminable" (Freud, 1937)).

Bisexuality is anchored in the narcissistic origins of psychosexuality and can be maintained throughout life by the immovable omnipotence of the same object; it is also inherited from the Oedipus complex and the enormous differentiation movement that it determines, establishing a firm Superego, sexual identifications and object choices.

McDougall (1988) also starts from the Freudian concept of bisexuality, adding that every child will want to possess the sexual organs of the man or the woman, endowed with their phantasmatic power, affirming that one of the most scandalous wounds for infantile megalomania is that inflicted by the obligation to accept our biological monosexuality. In the oedipal phase, with its dimension that is both homosexual and heterosexual, the child is forced to come to terms with the impossible desire to possess both parents, to belong to both sexes and to embody the two genital organs. For McDougall, the confusion these bisexual longings engender in the early organization of the psychosexual structure weighs upon many aspects of our adult life.

The Freudian psychic apparatus is organized around the notion of conflict, and sexuality is subordinated to conflict. Green (1973) in "El género neutro" [The neutral gender], illustrates how the psychic sex of the individual depends on how it is perceived and experienced by his father and mother, on their convergent or divergent desires towards the daughter, and the son towards his parents. This situation concludes in the fantasy of the primal scene, which will organize contradictory identifications. When conflict and fantasy do not contribute to the psyche's organization, the counterpart and complement of psychic bisexuality would be, as Green describes it, "the fantasy of the neutral gender, neither feminine nor masculine, dominated by an absolute primordial narcissism."

The presence or absence of a penis is distinctive in being symbolized. According to Green, there is a good reason to think that penis envy is not envy for that piece of flesh. Instead, it is what in fantasy confers power, being conferred by a parental wish.

Some countries, for example, Germany and Sweden, authorize parents to register their children at birth as of "indeterminate sex." This situation is yet another challenge for psychoanalysts. It was understandable that Freud found it difficult to harmonize the idea of biological bisexuality based on ideas about repression and the prevalence of the phallus for both sexes. For psychoanalysts of the 21st century, it is also a challenge. The object of sexual excess can generate deadly narcissistic breaks, producing a regression to pre-genital excitability, which can lead to a rupture (Laufer 1997).

The necessary search for identity in young people, which sometimes difficult to find, may become a basic privation, especially when there is no possibility of identification with the parental imagos. Therefore, the search for a framework of belonging can initiate an immense experience of anguish and pain. Becoming part of a group, a team, a protest cause, can become highly dangerous. The situation today leads young people into highly dangerous contexts (drug trafficking, murders incited by brainwashing) exposing the risk of being included in dangerous groups, or facing expulsion by authoritarian leaders. Suicide attempts are generally triggered after puberty by an adolescent's reaction to changes in the newly sexually mature body. The body is perceived as the enemy, and sometimes the death of the body seems to be the only recourse. These deadly disturbances expose the adolescent to the risk of losing the object and himself, generating situations that can lead to suicide or homicide without us knowing if the unconscious desire is to kill himself or their inner image of their parents. Unfortunately, we also see a high number of suicides in children today.

Today, there are different factors which produce a significant influence on children, adolescents, and adults: globalization, the immeasurable force of social networks, militant groups for the rights of children, the rights of women, the rights of numerous groups such as the LGTBQ, migrants, and many minority groups who do not feel represented or heard. The sense of belonging promised by these groups, means that they are faced with the difficulty of carrying an extremely fragile identity, especially when children or adolescents have experienced traumatic situations inside or outside the family, in environments that may have been excessively violent or excitable, generating sexual abuse, incest, or bodily harm, which may have left depressive marks, making it impossible for those children and adolescents to assemble identifications that fortify the self.

Cherchez la femme

The French expression meaning "seek the woman" comes from the novel by Alexander Dumas (1871), *Cherchez la femme, pardieu, cherchez la femme!* Referring to the fact that "in all cases, as soon as they bring me a report, I say, look for the woman!"

The phrase represents a cliché of detective literature: that no matter what the problem, a woman is often the cause of it. The term has come to be used to refer to explanations that inevitably have the same common root, regardless of the characteristics of the problem.

The interest generated by this statement is focused on this case, in which the woman will always appear as an accomplice in some unfair situation; it becomes a matter of looking for her, and for better or for worse, she will be found, emerging from the shadows, not knowing what the enigma with which man will find himself. This phrase was perpetuated in dozens of crime novels and film noir plots, attributing any distressing situation in the story to a woman in the shadows while provoking the leading actor to behave unreasonably in the eyes of those who thought they knew him. With the passage of time and their struggles, women have been able to prevent, in some way, being that object of perdition for men. Therefore, the phrase began later to resonate differently.

Cherchez la femme, then, charged a different dimension. When a man achieves success in politics, business, or his profession, it has been alluded to that it is mainly because a woman is behind him, guiding his destiny without which he would not reach the goal. This is how she seems to have been transforming, from the role of enigmatic sorceress, upsetting the most lucid minds, to elevating the man to positions of power without him realizing that he owed everything to her. Although, one fateful day, she would have to ask him to reflect on it.

Freud's prejudices concerning women had not impeded him from admiring Lou Andreas Salomé's comprehension, intelligence, intuition and capability. He consulted her on psychoanalytic issues, and also concerning his family, especially Anna. He invited Lou to stay in their house with her daughter. It was after Lou's stay in their home that Anna began her analysis, in fact, her "impossible" analysis with the father. Thus, Lou represented Anna as a model, both a thinker and a woman analyst. Although Lou died two years and a half before Freud, he recognized that her extraordinary qualities as an intellectual and the "exquisitely feminine" aspect in her intellectual work, the conjunction of the two qualities, femininity, and intellectual output, was significant. This is not only evident in Freud's discourse but may be also appreciated from our own perspective. The femininity inherent in Lou's intellectual work makes us think that she could situate herself in a desiring position with respect to love as well as to intellectual work and psychoanalysis (Abrevaya 2023).

Glocer Fiorini (2008) emphasizes the feminine enigma inherent to the origins to the finite time of life and to sexual difference. The basic misunderstanding stemming from this enigmatic condition is an equation of the feminine to the otherness.

The social revolution at the end of the 20th century brought about "the right to choose" for women, allowing them to become mothers or not. The repudiation of motherhood, which used to be considered by the psychoanalysts as an expression of the masculinity complex, became a feminist posture. Thus, in this sense, motherhood is no longer a privileged expression of femininity. The new types of families, such as those composed of single parents living with their children or those formed by parents of the same sex, is an impressive and vital change. These changes have shaken the basis of our perception and knowledge in terms of gender, sexuality, and motherhood.

Psychoanalysis is no stranger to the new discourses on women, femininity, and sexuality. The psychoanalyst's ideas of gender also permeate the transference relationship, even when they make no judgment about the patient's beliefs or ideologies. Knowledge is always partial and is generated from circumstances that are constantly changing (Haraway 2016). The search inside the female body is a claim to the knowledge of another universe, internal and very vast. It could be an option of displacement and discovery for the female collective, traditionally constrained by all civilizations, to their family and personal boundaries.

Twenty-first-century approaches show that the sex/gender system traverses culture and organizes society, with gender being a constitutive element of social relations and a primary form of power relations.

Perhaps, the centuries of submission have managed to make a mark, a footprint: we can identify this situation in many ways, reality shows us that is extremely difficult to eradicate. The patriarchy maintains its strength in such a way that it would explain a large portion of the great cruelties towards women. It is precisely why in practically no text will we find a similar allusion to men in the psychoanalytic sense intended to be given to the term.

Many women have died hoisting the flag of greater freedom and openness regarding their condition. We will have to reconsider ourselves then, if what a woman wants is so enigmatic, or being able to accept that there are infinite nuances between women and men that predominate in different ways under the influence of one's sex, the family, the social, the cultural, and above all by the desire of each human being, even though different environments make it hard to express.

We know that the capacity to feel deeply for another human being and for this feeling to be reciprocated is one of the most profound experiences that any of us can expect. This capacity for deep involvement with significant others depends on our earliest experiences. But the strength of angry, envious, and destructive feelings leads to a capacity for cruelty and damage. We all take pleasure in destruction, but our experiences in early life might also help us to bear this difficult aspect of ourselves avoiding a path leading to cruel and destructive actions. Is an excess of pleasure in human destructiveness the inverse proportion to the weakness of love of human commitment?

References

Abrevaya, E. (2023). *Femininity, Desire and Sublimation in Psychoanalysis. From the Melancholic to the Erotic*. London: Routledge.

André, J. (1994). *La sexualité féminine*. Que Sais-je?Paris: Presses Universitaires de France.

Aulagnier, P. (2003). *La violence de l'interprétation*. Fil rouge (le).Paris: Presses Universitaires de France.

Chabert, C. (2013). Perdre, abandonner, se trouver. In: *Les séparations: Victoires et catastrophes*. Le Carnet PSY. Toulouse: Éditions Érès.

Cournut-Janin, M. (1998). *Féminine et fèminitè*. Épîtres.Paris: Presses Universitaires de France.

Dumas, A. (1871). *Les Mohicans de Paris*. Paris: Michel Lévy Frères.

Faimberg, H. (2005). *The Telescoping of Generations: Listening to the Narcissistic Links between Generations*. New Library of Psychoanalysis. London: Routledge.

Freud, S. (1896) Fragments of letters with Fliess on bisexuality. *Etiology of Hysteria*, Sexuality in the etiology of neurosis.

Freud, S. (1905). *Tres ensayos de teoría sexual*, VII. Buenos Aires: Amorrortu editores, p. 109.

Freud, S. (1920). *Más allá del principio del placer*, XVIII. Buenos Aires: Amorrortu editores.

Freud, S. (1923). *La organización genital infantil (una interpretación de la teoría de la sexualidad)*, XIX. Buenos Aires: Amorrortu editores.

Freud, S. (1925). *Algunas consecuencias psíquicas de la diferencia anatómica entre los sexos*, XIX. Buenos Aires: Amorrortu editores, p. 259.

Freud, S. (1930a). *El malestar en la cultura*, XXI. Buenos Aires: Amorrortu editores, p. 57.

Freud, S. (1930b). *33 Conferencia "la feminidad"*, XXII. Buenos Aires: Amorrortu editores, p. 104.

Freud, S. (1937). *Análisis terminable e interminable*, XXIII. Buenos Aires: Amorrortu editores.

Glocer Fiorini, L. (2008). *Deconstructing the Feminine: Psychoanalysis, Gender and Theories of Complexity*. London: Routledge.

Godfrind, J. (2018). *From Bisexuality to the Feminine* in R. Jozef Perelberg (ed.), *Psychic Bisexuality: A British-French Dialogue*. London: Routledge.

Green, A. (1973). El género neutro. In: *Narcisismo de Vida, Narcisismo de Muerte*. Buenos Aires: Amorrortu editores.

Haraway, D. (2016). *Staying with the Trouble: Making Kin in the Chthulucene*. Durham, NC: Duke University Press.

Kahn, L. (2018). *L'écoute de l'analyste. De l'acte à la forme*. Paris: Presses Universitaires de France.

Kristeva, J. (1987). *Soleil noir: Dépression et mélancholie*. Paris: Gallimard.

Laplanche, J. (1988). *Three Destinations of the Enigmatic Message*. Conference held in Gramado, Brazil, 1–3 August.

Laufer, M. (1997). *Adolescent Breakdown and Beyond*. London: Routledge.

McDougall, J. (1966). *Theaters of the Mind: Illusion and Truth on the Psychoanalytic Stage*. London: Routledge.

McDougall, J. (1988). *Las mil y una caras de Eros, la sexualidad humana en busca de soluciones*. Buenos Aires: Paidos.

Volnovich, J.C. (2010). *The female figures that pass through the analysis among men Thematic Spaces Psychoanalysis*, Feminist Studies, and Gender. Psicomundo.com.

Winnicott, D. (1990). *The Maturational Processes and the Facilitating Environment: Studies in the Theory of the Emotional Development*. London: Routledge.

3   Of skin and of self-mutilation in adolescence

Martin Gauthier[1]

The physical maturation initiated with puberty brings about important changes in the adolescent's relationship with him or herself, with significant others, family and friends, and with the social community. The experience of the body and its representation enter major transformations with the unfolding sexual development: the whole body is the source of new experiences, sensations and pleasures. Erotogenicity, developed from infancy, has a special role in how the adolescent body will be inhabited and used in the process. Genital masturbation and all the various ways of seeking physical pleasures will be recruited in dealing with inner desires and emotional situations. When the adolescent is instead turning to self-mutilation, the analyst wonders how erotogenicity has failed or has been diverted. While more adolescents are turning to self-harm, the analyst also questions what makes this behaviour more prevalent nowadays.

Sarah and her self-mutilative behaviour

When I went to invite her to the office, she was already up, pacing the waiting room. The weather had been abnormally mild for early November, the mercury climbing for a few days above twenty degrees Celsius. I had been seeing Sarah for a few months. Usually dressed in dark clothes, she wore that afternoon a lighter t-shirt that highlighted the colourful tattoo covering her left arm. On her forearms, I could see whitish scars of scarifications that were slow to disappear. She was furious: "Have you seen what your friends around the corner are doing? In full summer temperature! It dries up, it dies, who cares! We get richer, the planet is burning and viva Christmas!".

And she left me to simmer for a few minutes imagining who these friends were and what they were doing to make her so upset. "*Comfortably numb,* as much as you are," she continued. I recognized the words of Pink Floyd, the band she was listening to and then discovered that my "friends around the corner" were the supermarket where Christmas decorations and accessories had appeared on 1 November as scheduled in the commercial timetable, without taking into account the weather and climate changes.

DOI: 10.4324/9781003380283-3

The parents of this 17-year old teenager, divorced and often quarrelling "for everything and especially over nothing", had presented a united front when their only child, "always so good in school and so bright", had decided not to return to class the previous winter. She had experienced occasional panic attacks and they had noticed her dietary restrictions, but they had ignored her self-mutilation, her experimental use of drugs and her occasional suicidal ideation. I had guessed her self-injury; she wore long-sleeved shirts even with the arrival of good weather. I learned the rest bit by bit in the midst of much anger and despair in the face of "a world that is going to its loss and doesn't care about it".

When I had directly questioned her about her self-mutilation on a sunny day, Sarah had revealed that she had been scratching or superficially cutting her forearms, although rarely her thighs, on a regular basis for the past two years. But she had quickly closed down, stating that she did not wish to speak about it further. Only later on, during a session following an argument that had led to cutting, did Sarah reluctantly add more details. She was, initially, using her fingernails, and later, any sharp object available. She could not remember how or why it had started: "I just had the idea". She would typically cut in the evening, when by herself in her room. It would "kind of empty my mind". As it had just happened, it could also take place following an argument, but rarely in school. "It grounds me; I feel calmer afterwards", she explained. "Everyone cuts", she said, and yet she had kept her behaviour hidden from her parents and close friends. She did not harbour suicidal thoughts when cutting but had had the idea of dying following angry fights with her parents (it would become clearer how those suicidal thoughts would play out some form of revenge against them).

During the November session (the time of the supermarket Christmas decorations), I had commented on Sarah's anger at the hypocrisy of the adults, and their way of covering up and blinding themselves to what was going on. Later on, I noticed that she was not covering her arms, a rare instance in my presence. I learned she had not cut for the past month and was feeling more comfortable if anyone noticed her scars. She had spoken about cutting to a friend and had discovered this friend was also cutting periodically. And more importantly, she added, it was the natural environment that needed attention as it was so poorly treated in "this crazy capitalistic society always racing for more". "There are sufferings that are not heard", I echoed.

Sarah's concerns for the environment had recently moved to the forefront after an initial period when I had largely heard about the uselessness of coming to therapy, which had only been accepted in order "to calm my parents down". She would describe various conflictual situations at home and with friends, blaming parents and peers, complaining about external decisions, with a sense of little personal power in her relationships. Feelings were poorly described with words and quickly discharged through acting, commonly by taking distance. Often overwhelmed, Sarah would find it easier to withdraw, listening to music (among which was Pink Floyd), scrolling on social media, or daydreaming (often replaying recent interactions). She saw herself having little influence on how her life was going and how she was feeling. The general state of the environment initially stimulated depressive anxieties which she could do little about. More recently, Sarah was more assertive in her expression of anger, targeting especially the general lack of concern towards nature and its exploitation. She had also started to become more active, involving herself in a community project. She was slowly beginning to value the contribution she could make and was supported by a group of peers welcoming her involvement.

Sarah, similarly to many adolescents who self-mutilate, had great difficulty tolerating her feelings and recognizing their nature by qualifying them through her words. Anger and anxiety were more manifest, but poorly differentiated and generally experienced as a tension in need to be expelled in order to avoid becoming too upset. Cutting one's skin had become a way to turn away from the emotional suffering, instead turning attention to the physical body and to pain (which was in fact better tolerated than emotional suffering – distinguishing *suffering* and *pain*, the former with its emotional/symbolic ramifications and the latter referring to the more concrete and non-symbolic physical pain). However the situation appeared to be evolving progressively. There were recent signs of a constructive movement outside and inside the therapeutic relationship.

A new emergence: adolescent self-mutilation

The self-injurious behaviours to which I am drawing attention in Sarah's presentation, are generally defined as the deliberate and direct alteration or destruction of body tissues, without danger to life or conscious suicidal intent.[2] These are of a different quality to the injuries presented in psychosis, where very serious situations can exist (actual castrations, enucleations or amputations), in autism spectrum disorder, in epilepsy, in substance abuse or in children suffering from an intellectual handicap. This definition also excludes behaviours culturally, or sub-culturally, accepted, which also involve deliberate alteration of the body, such as piercing, tattooing, body art or plastic surgery. It is however interesting to note how much current Western culture makes significant use of the skin as an expressive medium. We will return later to this observation, considering the cultural importance given to the skin and the significant prevalence of self-mutilation among adolescents.

There are many teenagers who self-harm and international epidemiological studies have reported an increased prevalence for the past 25 years (De Sene Moreira et al., 2020; Cybulski et al., 2021; Mercado et al., 2017). From being a rarer observation 40 years ago (Mansell Pattison & Kahan, 1983), self-mutilation has become a common condition among teenagers. Indeed, adolescence generally constitutes the period of emergence of these behaviours which can be limited in time (Louppe, 2001) or extend into adulthood.

Variable rates (roughly from one out of ten teenagers to four out of ten) have been reported from samples of adolescents in their community, while these rates double in samples of adolescents in clinical settings. Most commonly, self-harm takes the form of one or more superficial cuts (scarifications) to the skin of the upper arm and forearm, on the side opposite to the dominant hand, performed with a sharp object, but there may also be bites, shocks, burns, stings or pinches. Any skin surface can be affected, but it is usually a place that can be covered with clothing, and therefore not exposed. Much more rarely encountered is the direct attack on the genitals or the breasts, which raises more openly the problem of the erotic body and sexual identity. Sometimes, more rarely too, words or phrases are engraved on the skin, like another teenager who concealed from her environment that she had been raped a few months previously, until her social worker could decipher the word 'rape' within the succession of small cuts that she repeated on her forearm. Or another adolescent boy who engraved on his abdomen, among many scratches, the name of the girlfriend with whom he had recently broken up.

Typically self-harm does not overtly worry adolescents and it is hence underreported. It appears slightly more prevalent in girls than boys, but adolescent girls are also more inclined to seek help and are more represented in clinical settings. Self-injury is often discovered by an adult of the entourage who will worry about it, concerned in particular about suicidal risk (which is in fact higher in young people who self-harm without being a direct consequence of the behaviour itself, but a result of the underlying pathology). Or it is observed by a professional during a consultation for other reasons, especially because the scars remain visible for a long time. It was the case with Sarah, who did not raise spontaneously the issue of her self-mutilation, was initially unwilling to speak about it, and continued to hide it for a while.

Pain is generally not an issue in the discourse of those adolescents either. Rather, they generally insist on the calming and relieving character of their gesture when an internal tension becomes unbearable. They find it difficult to qualify this internal tension; different feelings or outlines of feelings are blurred together, typically with an element of anxiety and anger/hostility. Physical pain, as Sarah did explain, drives out inner suffering; it makes tension disappear. The primary gain of the self-injury appears personal and of an economical order, for the management of an ill-qualified internal quantity. The emotional self-regulatory function stands out. Over time, the scarifications can progress to becoming the result of repetitive, compulsive or automatic gestures done for personal homeostasis, without manifest thinking.

At a secondary level, various uses can be made of the self-harm behaviour itself within the teens' closer relationships. For example, an adolescent attacked her mother by exhibiting the scars of self-harm during an argument, wanting to show her how incompetent she was as a mother, and subsequently rejecting any movement of maternal solicitude in her direction. Her mother would become upset and self-accusatory for her daughter's predicament, and the latter would see an added confirmation that her mother was only concerned with herself. With Sarah, hiding her self-mutilation and remaining isolated with her suffering were used for some time as additional proofs that her analyst was useless and could not help her.

When a deeper clinical exploration is possible, an heterogeneous group of adolescents is discovered and there should be no question of bringing them all under the same metapsychological organization. Nor could their verbalizations about their behaviour and its effects be reduced under a single entity (Lindgren, Wikander, Marklund & Molin, 2022). Nevertheless, among the more concerning adolescents are those whose mental functioning gives a central place to acting over reflecting, and where a personal psychic space is poorly established. The puberty crisis seems to have led to a developmental breakdown (Laufer & Laufer, 1984). The power of the object remains dominant, in the maze of pirouettes to free oneself from anxieties of passivity, intrusion or abandonment. When emotions are too great, the threat of passivity is magnified, and self-mutilation offers an active means of claiming some agency and power on the body (and the object responsible for the affective experience).[3]

The past and present history of those more disturbed teenagers is often coloured by ill-conceived traumas and disruptions. The ruptures in their continuity – these cuts – have an echo at the internal level where structurally, splitting prevails and blocks the possibilities of elaboration. Losses remain unmourned. Overflows and voids coexist, with regressive falls, noisy or silent. These adolescents often complain about their current objects; they may want the analyst to intervene on their behalf in a concrete way, but rarely do they express an explicit wish for help concerning the self-harm. They do not want to be joined on this territory; they hold onto the emotional self-regulatory solution they have fabricated. It is experienced as helping to keep oneself together in a self-sufficient way. The risk of depending on an other appears too great. Expelling the tension and the object is a more expedient, safer avenue. They work hard at staying away from thinking about bad or upsetting memories, hence also avoiding any closeness which could evoke those thoughts.[4] Their skin can become like a parchment full of signs which they claim to be senseless, in no need of being read.

The battery of erotogenicity

The way the self-mutilative adolescent treats his or her own body deserves closer attention. It is tempting to quickly move to a symbolic level and associate such destructive gestures against the self to guilt and punishment, to a masochistic need, or to a melancholic movement protecting the object and denying loss. These deeper symbolic meanings can eventually emerge and play a significant role depending on the individual and his or her developmental path, but at first, with a significant number of self-mutilative teenagers, the symbolic level is not available or poor. The qualification of their emotional charge is limited, words are inadequate when it comes to feelings, the affective range and tolerance are narrow. The clinician needs to work initially at facilitating the qualification of emotional experiences, but he faces a resistance from the patient at letting him or her move closer to the emotional distress. To the contrary, the adolescent is not only cutting his skin, but also cutting away from any other who could assist him with his suffering. Instead of investing the relationship, a strong current of counter-investment (Cournut, 1989) is observed when it comes to needing the object. With the great transformations of puberty and adolescence, it questions the development of erotogenicity and the auto-erotic use of the skin in relation to narcissism and the expansion of the ego.

When it was conceptualized by Freud (1914), erotogenicity (or erogeneity) designated the sexual excitability of a part of the body, or more generally, the general property of the body to be a source of "sexually exciting stimuli". The notion was extended from the genitals to the whole body, and it varied quantitatively from one area to another. The concept was defined with the introduction of narcissism and Freud postulated a close relation between the investment of libido in the ego and erotogenicity.[5] The model of object libido fixation in transference neuroses found an equivalent with the stasis of ego libido in actual neuroses, notably in hypochondria. The focus was on economic considerations, the mental apparatus being recognized as "first and foremost a device designed for mastering excitations which would otherwise be felt as distressing or would have pathogenic effects" (Freud, 1914, p. 85). This economical perspective of the mental apparatus remained present when Freud (1920) addressed again the issue of trauma after the First World War and introduced the death drive. The focus on the quantitative factor continued to be central in the testamentary considerations of "Analysis Terminable and Interminable" (Freud, 1937).

Since the initial conceptualization, the evolution in the metapsychological conceptions of the drives and the ego has allowed a new perspective on the crossroad of erotogenicity. A new epigenesis has emerged, giving a greater role to its development in the relational bosom. The focus thus continued to move away from a constitutional basis towards the relational construction of the erogenous body in the interactions with caregivers. Freud (1895) had first taken that direction when he used Charcot's notion of *hysterogenic zone* to speak of an *atypical hysterogenic zone* while exploring Elisabeth von R's pains to her right thigh, eventually extending the concept and conceptualizing an *erotogenous zone*. The sexual responsiveness was recognized as determined by the subject's history and not by anatomy or by some constitutional defect, which was Charcot's explanation for hysteria.

The post-Freudian emphasis on object relations and on the early foundations of the mental apparatus has continued to move erotogenicity away from being a given towards being a complex construct. In the wake of the idea of a development of the drives starting with an initial qualification of the somatic excitation (Green, 1975), erotogenicity can be conceived as the result of the initial linking of libido by the growing ego, initially the body ego, with the support of the primary object, under the aegis of the pleasure principle. It builds the foundations of the erotogenous body and of the ego on the traces left by the early interactive experiences. With the initial process of mentalisation and subjective appropriation, excitement takes shape and gives shape. The body thus starts to be symbolized and it progressively belongs to the subject through its erogenous qualification. The work of representation and erotogenicity form two founding functions of the unconscious ego, faithful to its generative potential.

This erotogenous body has an individual geography, shaped by the traces of the early relations. At the heart of the absolute dependence and helplessness of the little human, in the multimodal exchanges with the primary object,[6] the map of a first indistinct mother-child body is drawn from which the child's own body will gradually emerge, as well as those of mother and father. This whole process involves the ego in becoming, imperatively supported by the auxiliary ego of the object, with its own erotogenicity. Above all, it summons the complex process of linking that we call symbolization. André Green (2005) spoke of the psyche as "the relation between two bodies, one of which is absent".

Various facets of the early relationships and the birth of psychic life have been emphasized by different psychoanalytic authors, for example the maternal holding and mirroring (Winnicott) or the maternal containing and reverie (Bion), to name but two. What the notion of erotogenicity brings to the fore is the importance of the libidinal source of psychic life and its appropriation. In each individual development, this source cannot be taken for granted constitutionally and it continues to evolve through life. Erotogenicity is the battery of the self, its converter of raw excitement into libidinal energy at the service of the ego. The investment of the ego passes through the erotogenicity of its contents and its functioning, through the erotogenicity of the bodily ego at its foundations. The ego is first of all a bodily ego, as Freud (1923) emphasized. And this bodily ego is inherently erotogenous.

Self-mutilation places the skin at the foreground. It highlights its limits and its possible transformations. The French psychoanalyst Didier Anzieu (1985, 1993) has brought attention to the skin and to what he calls the *skin-ego* (*le moi-peau*). He emphasized the basic function of the skin, both at an organic and at an imaginary level, protecting the subject's individuality while being the first tool and locus of exchange with others. Recognizing how much the psychic apparatus rests on the support of the physical body and of the social body (initially represented by the primary object), he postulated the importance of a skin-ego, a metaphor at the crossroads of fantasies and interactive exchanges. Physical container and interface of communication, the skin separates the inside from the outside; it becomes the basis for the psychic envelope of the ego. As mentioned earlier, Freud (1923) had opened the way when he wrote: "The ego is first and foremost a bodily ego; it is not merely a surface entity, but is itself the projection of a surface".[7] Winnicott (1988) spoke later of the imaginative elaboration of physical function and the importance of the psyche-soma integration. Esther Bick (1968, 1986) also described the importance of a first skin (similar to Anzieu's skin-ego) and the possible defensive development of a second-skin formation when the primary dependence on the object is too precarious.

Erotogenicity is a dimension that goes back to the infant and his or her interactions. But it designates a property of the ego interface always at work in the actuality of the object relations. It is anchored in the present of the relationship to the body and to the object; it is an active, open process. At this interface, erotogenicity refers to the ego's ability to channel the excitatory load towards its own functioning. But there is always a risk of exceeding a critical threshold where the linking capacities are overwhelmed and where trauma begins (opening another territory where other laws prevail, beyond the pleasure principle). Self-mutilation opens a dike.

The notion of erotogenicity can be extended towards the associated concept of auto-erotism. Freud (1905) borrowed the latter term from the British sexologist Havelock Ellis to describe those situations where the subject obtains a sexual satisfaction from his own body, without turning to an object. His first example was thumb-sucking, with the child's lips being the first erotogenic zone and the thumb a second one (of an inferior order, Freud said, as compared to the breast or its substitute). The concept of auto-erotism has also evolved over time as greater attention was given to the role of the object in the early stages of mental life. A useful distinction for the purpose of this discussion is drawn between auto-erotism and auto-sensuality.

In auto-erotism, the movement *auto*, towards oneself, constitutes a positive developmental step when it signs an appropriation, an increasing ownership. It demonstrates a new mental capacity for pleasure initiated by the self. Something of the object responsible for the previous experience of pleasure, and something of the experience of pleasure itself have been internalized. The object is retained, initially in a proto-symbolic and eventually in a symbolic form detached from its concreteness, opening up progressively the field of fantasy. In this perspective, auto-erotism is constructed in the relationship with the object: it is not without an object, it is the path of a mental object. In fact, the process becomes conflictual when the external object is reluctant to give up its exclusivity in the gratification of pleasures (Abraham, 1978). This auto-erotic movement, directly associated to the shaping of erotogenicity, plays a crucial role in the constitution of the ego, in the constantly renewed integrative process called narcissism. Taking pleasure in one's own functioning is the cornerstone and the cement of one's personal space.

Thus, in the proposed definition of auto-erotism, the object remains fundamental but the subject has internalized it on his or her own internal scene. On the other hand, different authors have described auto-sensory and self-calming behaviours (Szwec, 1998), where the overt activity serves to counter-invest the object, or even to disinvest it. The relationship with the object is not maintained but evacuated, the discharge reflecting an inability to deal internally with the excitation created in contact with it. Contrary to auto-erotism, auto-sensuality designates an activity, often repetitive, compulsive or addictive, dissociated from the object, in a somewhat close system creating and mastering its own excitation. The vitality of the internal representation of the object and of the link with it differentiates the autoerotic from the auto-sensory as the external behaviour may be similar (although the auto-sensory activity is typically more extreme, exhausting).

It is worth mentioning here an observation Winnicott (1953) made in his famous paper on transitional objects and transitional phenomena. As an example, he described two brothers X and Y. X was never a thumb-sucker and had a rabbit as a *comforter* that "never had the quality of a true transitional object"[8] as it was never more important than the mother, while Y sucked his thumb and elected a blanket as a *soother*, a true transitional object. In the complex passage from the external object as the exclusive source of satisfaction to the internal object and the internal agency of the self, Winnicott emphasized the importance of the intermediate area offered by transitional phenomena. The auto-erotic movement partakes in this process. The mother who does not allow the creation of a transitional object more important than herself is blocking auto-erotism (and the symbolization process that accompanies it). Self-calming behaviours can eventually be used to fill the void and give the illusion of self-sufficiency.

An economical and anti-metaphorical solution

As stated earlier, self-mutilation can evoke spontaneously the idea of an attack on the self, based on a guilty, masochistic or melancholic underlying movement. The concern for a suicidal gesture follows this logic. Those dynamics can play an implicit role for some adolescents (Sarah's treatment later on involved the working through of a melancholic core in which she protected her primary objects by blaming herself), but a majority of them present initially a more direct need to discharge inner tensions that are poorly differentiated. In this regard, teenagers who self-mutilate unveil a special use of their skin where a dysfunction of erotogenicity can be recognized. At an age where the major physical changes of puberty impose a new geography and mapping of the bodily ego, they do not or cannot call on the erotogenicity of the body in their distress and choose instead a kind of "shutting off" or "black out" (expressions often used by teenagers who self-mutilate when asked about its effects), cutting away from the erotogenous source.

Increasing external stimulation can be sought out as a response to an increased internal tension. For instance, when distressed, some adolescents will use physical exercise, loud music, or genital masturbation as external stimulations bringing relief, if not pleasure. There are quite a number of ways by which the erogenous charge of the body is called upon in order to deal with an emotional tension until it is possible to qualify it and work it through. However, in this regard, self-mutilation is a paradoxical increase in the stimulation of the skin in order to diminish the erotogenous charge and return to a neutral state. The emotional charge is not transformed but evacuated, with a parallel impoverishment in symbolic content and life. A kind of anti-metaphorical solution is used, the economical factor prevailing over any possible qualification.

Clinicians working with psychosomatic patients have described such anti-metaphorical movements (Marty, 1998; Szwec, 1998). De M'Uzan (2003) spoke of slaves of quantity (*esclaves de la quantité*) around the example of a severe masochistic patient. Major traumas, such as the experience of concentration camps during the Second World War, have also been implicated in generating such defences (Grubrich-Simitis, 1984, 2010) but they have also been associated with pathological mourning (Abraham & Torok, 1978). Without the circulation of an open symbolization process, erotogenicity comes up against a resistance that blocks its rich deployment. Splitting can prevail and maintains the subjective non-appropriation of the body, mutilated in its erotogenicity. The basis for a rich deployment is the relation to the object and this is what the clinician will want to remain very sensitive to.

Any discharge is a source of pleasure, so much so that Freud found it difficult to conceive of pleasure other than in terms of discharge. Any solution to a conflict, no matter how lame, allows a relaxation, even if only partial. "What can you offer me instead of the solution I found for myself?", seems to tell these teenagers view us with suspicion. More so, their self-injurious solution is now popularized on websites, exposed on television, in the cinema or in music videos, and it is contagious, as we know from psychiatric units and penitentiaries. So what do we have to offer? To feel the pain rather than evacuate it? And how is this done, and what does it lead to?

All these aspects, from experiencing pain and qualifying it to working through internal emotions and conflicts, cannot be considered in a solipsistic fashion: the object is crucial in their development. The other constitutes the *space of resonance* for the self (Schneider, 2002). The work of Winnicott and Ferenczi have emphasized the role of trauma when the object fails at providing that space. Green has proposed to view the psyche as taking place in the internal frame created by the negative hallucination of the primary object.

It is a complex question that these adolescents raise when they wonder how the pleasure of discharging can be replaced by pleasure obtained by containing and transforming. Freud offered some metapsychological grounds when he differentiated the Nirvana principle (the reduction of excitation to zero, in the footsteps of the introduction of the death drive) from the pleasure principle and the reality principle. The pleasure principle establishes its domination through libidinal linking of the drive, which involves necessarily the object. The field of symbolisation is an expansion of object-relations. In the process, the maturation of the ego holds a gradient of tension made possible by what Rosenberg (1991) called a *life-protecting masochism* (*masochisme gardien de la vie*) in his reading of Freud's primary erotogenic masochism (Freud, 1924). Taking pleasure in tolerating some tension is the basis for developing an internal space which will be growing along with new experiences associated to the auto-erotic fantasies symbolisation makes possible. On the contrary, masochistic defences are raised when the experience of helplessness is excessive and anxieties too poorly qualified (Rosenberg, 1991; Gauthier, 1994).

The emphasis placed on the role of the object has importance in the here and now of the therapeutic relationship with teenagers who self-harm. The closest violence may appear to be in the concrete gesture itself, in the attack on the skin and the body, and its underlying symbolic meaning; but in a silent way, it is also a direct attack on the relation to the object whom the subject does not turn to and cuts away from. The mutilation concerns the relationship. Violence resides in the breaking of relational continuity. The concrete cut hides and reveals a more insidious and serious one at the relational level (with the history of previous relationships each adolescent will unravel during treatment).

This is my experience in the treatment of these self-mutilating adolescents: it is essential to focus on establishing a bond with them and to tactfully (Ferenczi, 1928) address the self-injury as a way of cutting away from that bond. Their pathological self-regulation of internal tensions passes through a silent disinvestment, and this disinvestment needs to be recognized in order to explore its dynamics and history. In parallel, a new space is created to contain together and work at qualifying the affects, instead of evacuating them. The session can become a new symbolic skin, an expanding envelope. It is also a surface of contact and an interface with the analyst. The therapeutic bond in turn provokes affective reactions which put to the test the developing relationship. Roussillon (2010; 2015) hence spoke of the object as needing to be symbolized while helping in its symbolisation (*l'objet à symboliser et pour symboliser*).

Linking and symbolizing will however raise resistances of various strengths and the elaboration of those resistances, with the anxieties attached to them, can be a lengthy endeavour. Fundamentally, the counter-investment nested in the anti-metaphorical presentation needs to be addressed. When disinvesting stops prevailing, the symbolic dimensions, in particular the sexual aspects, of the self-injury can become available. The self-injury can then more easily be considered as an attack on the adolescent (sexual) body, a body that does violence in itself given the lack of control over it and the difficulty owning it.

In fact, the counter-investment is only one side of the coin. It is a powerful defence against the over-cathexis of the object. It is the need to free oneself from the power of the object that makes disinvestment so necessary. The battle at the level of the skin speaks about the difficulty in establishing a solid enough narcissism in the commerce with the object. In this perspective, the mutilated skin also represents unconsciously that of the object, confused with that of the subject who struggles to differentiate himself or herself. The violence applied to the skin reveals the difficulties, past and present, in this process of self-object differentiation (and in owning one's erotogenicity and auto-erotism). A lively and creative separation appears conflictual. The support of the object in the process is not established.

Sarah's self-injury diminished and gradually disappeared while she progressively allowed her analyst to move closer. She was initially very reluctant to make any connection between her self-mutilation and her therapeutic relationship, wishing to consider them as unrelated. Her ecological preoccupations, especially for the destructive forces at play in the lack of care for the environment, slowly opened the door to considering her anxieties about her own ambivalent feelings and her way of dealing and not dealing with them. The recognition of her reparative gestures (such as her involvement in her community and its reception by her peers, as well as in her analysis) played an important role in building a more constructive representation of herself while making possible to address the more destructive aspects without despair or flight (Winnicott, 1963). But in the first place, it was important to address the counter-investment at play in the self-injury. The latter was not only like making a hole in her own mental envelope, evacuating any possible qualification of what she was feeling; but it was also a silent attack of the therapeutic link the analyst offered. At a wider level, it was a retreat from the social group, which she slowly constructed new links with, as her reparative gestures were welcomed.

Concluding with a cultural perspective

Sarah initially presented with a decision to not return to school, refusing the path her parents and society were tracing for her and denouncing how the adult world was functioning. She was very concerned by environmental degradation, with its (initially unrecognized) resonance with her past and its frightening foreboding. She was connected with the world and with her peers through her social preoccupations, yet disconnected in her private suffering. Self-mutilation was a hidden symptom that gave paradoxically access to her own movement of disinvestment. Bringing the latter to the fore opened a speaking space for a symbolic qualification of the feelings and underlying conflicts which mutilated her when they were blindly expelled. Her body claimed a fuller erotogenicity and her auto-erotism explored more creative ways of cutting and separating. Her analysis was a self-appropriative endeavour.

Ida Bauer, known as Dora in Freud's famous case history, was Sarah's age when she started treatment in mid-October 1900 (Mahony, 1996). She saw Freud for two and half months, ending abruptly the analysis she had started at her father's request (in Sarah's case, her parents had joined forces). She complained of somatic symptoms (coughing spells, fainting, convulsion, aphonia) and had written a suicidal note. She was not self-mutilating but her body was central in her presentation, in an era when sexual repression was important for women especially. The case history gave a first dynamic explanation of how conversion symptoms unfold progressively.

More than a century later, Dora's case history remains an illustration of how Freud practised psychoanalysis and the use he made of dreams. With hindsight, many aspects of the case betray its historical determinism, starting with how prevalent the diagnosis of conversion hysteria was at the time. The clinical presentation of adolescents and the diagnostic classifications have evolved since. This raises questions about the historical and sociological factors playing a role in the aetiology and in the expression of psychological distress in adolescence.

Could current social and cultural factors be associated to the increased prevalence of self-harm among young people? How is society influencing the form taken by the adolescent distress and its interpretation? This query opens up a larger reflection on the relationship between the individual and society, and more specifically the adolescent and the social group he or she is growing in. It invites us to consider the interdependence of the individual and the group.

A distinction was initially made between self-mutilatory behaviours that are socially integrated (linking the individual to its culture or to a sub-culture) and the private ones (Green, 1997) without such an explicit social connection and without symbolic representations. In the socialized paradigm, a form is given to the need to feel part of the group, while offering simultaneously a way of appropriating the body and oneself. The individual dances with the group. The isolated self-injurious adolescent performs his or her difficulty joining the dance. This performance leaves a visible mark on the skin, a reminder for the individual, a hidden sign at the interface with the social body. By progressively becoming part of the self-injurious practice, the analyst wants to make it significant and to re-establish a connection between the individual and the group.

The high prevalence of self-mutilation is a sign of distress among contemporary teenagers.[9] On the one hand, this chapter has wanted to emphasize the importance of the skin and of erotogenicity for the individual at all age, but in a special way for the adolescent facing the task of owning the transformations of his or her body. On the other hand, society has also been evolving rapidly in the past decades, with the growth of digital technology and internet, greater international mobility and major changes in the family structure. At such times of transformation, with new social uncertainties and threats, such as the ecological crisis dear to Sarah, what support is society offering to teenagers in order to help them dance with the group?

In parallel with self-mutilation, different social practices, such as tattooing, piercing or plastic surgery, have become popular and also place an emphasis on the skin. While technological progress allows increased distance in communications and modify human relationships, could there be a need to return to the skin in order to rekindle the basis of the skin-ego and of erotogenicity in order to own more fully the connection with oneself and with others? Self-mutilation would however be a failed attempt unless it is heard and symbolized. At that condition, the erotogenous body can develop its astonishing possibilities of creative connections. In their unique ways, in their unique era, contemporary adolescents remain "engaged in the perpetual human task of keeping inner and outer reality separate yet interrelated" (Winnicott, 1971, p. 3).

Notes

1 Martin Gauthier M.D. is a Child and Adolescent Psychiatrist and a Training Analyst in private practice in Montreal, Canada. For 35 years, he treated children, adolescents and their families at the Montreal Children's Hospital, and taught at McGill University. He is a former President of the Canadian Psychoanalytic Society and of the Société psychanalytique de Montréal, as well as a former North-American representative on the Board of the International Psychoanalytic Association.
2 The definition used here is of *non-suicidal self-injury* (NSSI) – deliberate, self-inflicted destruction of body tissue without suicidal intent and for purposes not socially sanctioned – adopted by most researchers within Canada and the United States. It fits with the condition proposed in the DSM-5 under Non-suicidal Self-Injury. In contrast, the term *deliberate self-harm* (DSH) is frequently employed as a more encompassing reference to self-injurious behaviours both with and without suicidal intent that have non-fatal outcomes. This latter term is used predominantly within European countries and in Australia (Muehlenkamp et al., 2012).
3 By nature, affects are first experienced passively. André Green (1973) defined affect as a bodily and psychic experience, in which the first is the condition of the second. He wrote: "Here the body is acted and not agent, passive and not active, spectator and not actor. The body is not the subject of an action but the object of a passion. [...] Affect is a gaze on the moved body" (Green, 1973, p. 221, my translation). Green's ideas on affects were published in English in 1999.
4 Higher avoidance was found to be a main predictor of future self-injury in young adolescent girls by Gromatsky et al. (2020). When the link to others is present from the outset in the more hysterical mode of a superficial identification with comrades or desirable figures who self-harm, it appears easier to establish a therapeutic relationship, the disinvestment being less significant.
5 "We can decide to regard erotogenicity as a general characteristic of all organs and may then speak of an increase or decrease of it in a particular part of the body. For every such change in the erotogenicity of the organs there might then be a parallel change of libidinal cathexis in the ego" (Freud, 1914, p. 84).
6 With Bollas (2000), the "primary object" refers to a construct often called "mother". The primary caretaker is at the heart of this representation but the whole experience of the first relations partakes in the construction.
7 Freud, 1923, p. 26.
8 Winnicott, 1971, p. 8.
9 From a group perspective, it can also be postulated that teenagers express with their own means a more general social distress in the present culture, along with the difficulty turning this pain into a more manifest and organized resistance. The same logic applies to the eco-anxiety experienced by Sarah and many young people in society, although more actions are now generated on that front.

References

Anzieu, D. (1985). *Le Moi-Peau*. Paris: Dunod.
Anzieu, D. (1993). Autistic phenomena and the skin ego. *Psychoanalytic Inquiry* 13(1): 42–48.

Abraham, N. (1978). Le 'crime' de l'introjection. In: Abraham, N. & Torok, M., *L'écorce et le noyau*, pp. 123–131. Paris: Aubier Flammarion.

Abraham, N. & Torok, M. (1978). Deuil ou mélancolie. In: *L'écorce et le noyau*, pp. 259–275. Paris: Aubier Flammarion.

Bick, E. (1968). The experience of the skin in early object-relations. *International Journal of Psychoanalysis* 49(2): 84–486.

Bick, E. (1986). Further considerations on the function of the skin in early object relations: Findings from infant observation integrated into child and adult analysis. *British Journal of Psychotherapy* 2(4): 92–299.

Bollas, C. (2000) *Hysteria*. Oxford: Routledge.

Cournut, J. (1989). Les deux contre-investissements de l'excitation. *Nouvelle Revue de psychanalyse* 39: 1–94.

Cybulski, L. et al. (2021). Temporal trends in annual incidence rates for psychiatric disorders and self-harm among children and adolescents in the UK, 2003–2018. *BMC Psychiatry* 21(229).

De M'Uzan, M. (2003). Slaves of quantity. *The Psychoanalytic Quarterly* 72(3): 711–725.

De Sene Moreira, E. et al.(2020). Self-mutilation among adolescents: an integrative review of the literature. *Ciência & Saude Coletiva* 25(10): 3945–3954.

Ferenczi, S. (1928). The Elasticity of Psycho-Analytic Technique. *Final Contributions to the Problems and Methods of Psychoanalysis*. London: Karnac Books, pp. 87–101.

Freud, S. (1895). Studies in Hysteria. *S.E.* II, pp. 3–319.

Freud, S. (1905). Three Essays on Sexuality. *S.E.* VII, pp. 135–245.

Freud, S. (1914). On Narcissism: An Introduction. *S.E.* XIV, pp. 73–102.

Freud, S. (1920). Beyond The Pleasure Principle. *S.E.* XVIII, pp. 7–64.

Freud, S. (1923). The Ego and the Id. *S.E.* XIX, pp. 12–66.

Freud, S. (1924). The Economic Problem of Masochism. *S.E.* XIX, pp. 159–170.

Freud, S. (1937). Analysis Terminable and Interminable. *S.E.* XXIII, pp. 216–253.

Gauthier, M. (1994). De l'objet secourable: désaide et masochisme. In: J. Laplanche et al., *Colloque international de psychanalyse*. Paris: Presses Universitaires de France, pp. 57–68.

Green, A. (1975). The analyst, symbolization and absence in the analytic setting (on changes in analytic practice and analytic experience) – In memory of D. W. Winnicott. *International Journal of Psychoanalysis* 56: 1–22.

Green, A. (1973). *Le discours vivant*. Paris: Presses Universitaires de France.

Green, A. (1997). *On Private Madness*. Madison, WI: International Universities Press.

Green, A. (1999). *The Fabric of Affect in the Psychoanalytic Discourse*. London & New York: The New Library of Psychoanalysis.

Green, A.(2005). *Play and Reflection in Donald Winnicott's Writings*. London: Karnac Books.

Gromatsky, M.A. et al. (2020). Prospective prediction of first onset of nonsuicidal self-injury in adolescent girls. *Journal of the American Academy of Child and Adolescent Psychiatry* 59(9): 1049–1057.

Grubrich-Simitis, I. (1984). From concretism to metaphor – thoughts on some theoretical and technical aspects of the psychoanalytic work with children of Holocaust survivors. *Psychoanalytic Study of the Child*, 39: 301–319.

Grubrich-Simitis, I. (2010). Reality testing in place of interpretation: a phase in psychoanalytic work with descendants of Holocaust survivors. *Psychoanalytic Quarterly* 79(1): 37–69.

Lindgren, B-M., Wikander, T., Marklund, I.N. & Molin, J. (2022). A necessary pain: a literature review of young people's experiences of self-harm. *Issues in Mental Health Nursing* 43(2): 154–163.

Laufer, M. & Laufer, M.E. (1984). *Adolescence and Developmental Breakdown.* New Haven: Yale University Press.

Louppe, A. (2001). Automutilations transitoires à l'adolescence. *Revue française de psychanalyse* 65: 463–475.

Mahony, P. (1996). *Freud's Dora: A Psychoanalytic, Historical, and Textual Study.* New Haven: Yale University Press.

Mansell Pattison, E. & Kahan, J. (1983). The Deliberate Self-Harm Syndrome. *American Journal of Psychiatry* 140(7): 867–872.

Marty, P. (1998). *Les mouvements individuels de vie et de mort.* Paris: Payot.

Mercado, M.C. et al. (2017). Trends in emergency department visits for nonfatal self-inflicted injuries among youth aged 10 to 24 years in the United States, 2001–2015. *Journal of the American Medical Association* 318(19): 1931–1933.

Muehlenkamp, J.J., Claes, L., Havertape, L. & Plener, P.L. (2012). International prevalence of adolescent non-suicidal self-injury and deliberate self-harm. *Child and Adolescent Psychiatry and Mental Health* 6, Art.10.

Rosenberg, B. (1991). *Masochisme mortifère et masochisme gardien de la vie.* Monographies de la Revue française de psychanalyse. Paris: Presses Universitaires de France.

Roussillon, R. (2010). La fonction symbolisante de l'objet. In: Golse, B. & Roussillon, R., *La naissance de l'objet.* Paris: Presses Universitaires de France, pp. 127–154.

Roussillon, R. (2015). An introduction to the work of primary symbolization. *International Journal of Psychoanalysis* 96(3): 583–594.

Schneider, M. (2002). La souffrance psychique. In: Y. Michaud (ed.), *Qu'est-ce que la vie psychique?* Paris: Odile Jacob, pp. 141–155.

Szwec, G. (1998). *Les galériens volontaires.* Paris: Presses Universitaires de France.

Winnicott, D.W. (1953). Transitional objects and transitional phenomena. *International Journal of Psychoanalysis* 34(2): 89–97.

Winnicott, D.W. (1963). The development of the capacity for concern. *Bulletin of the Menninger Clinic* 27(4): 167–176.

Winnicott, D.W. (1971). *Playing and Reality.* London: Pelican Books.

Winnicott, D.W. (1988). *Human Nature.* London: Free Association Books.

4 The turbulence of puberty in an uncertain world

Virginia Ungar

The starting point of this chapter is a quote from Bion, who points out that the latent element during latency is a certain *emotional turbulence*. He goes on to say that,

> when the quiet, cooperative, nicely behaved boy or girl becomes noisy, rebellious and troublesome, the emotional upheaval rapidly ceases to be limited by the physiological boundaries of what we call John, Jack, Jill, or Jean in his or her corporeal frame.
>
> (Bion, 1977)

He then refers to some drawings by Leonardo da Vinci of "water swirling in turmoil, of hair in disorder," and quotes Milton's "Paradise Lost," with the aim of allowing readers to evoke similar images from their own scientific, artistic or religious heritage to recall a time in mental life marked by a sort of emotional turbulence similar to that addressed by psychoanalysts. Bion is convinced that psychoanalysts should retrieve those periods of mental turmoil that found them in their most turbulent form. His description denotes our feelings and lessons learned from experiencing sessions with adolescents under his guidance.

In analytic practice, adolescent turbulence rattles the analyst's infantile structures, as this turmoil is felt very intensely in respect to the analyst's countertransference. It is quite difficult to maintain the analytical attitude when the patient is more inclined to action than to introspection. In these situations, patients are apparently uninterested in knowing what is going on in their inner world, though if one manages to find a motivation – not a reason, nor a motive – sessions with young patients undergoing puberty can be a fascinating experience.

Donald Meltzer (1993) has made significant contributions to the understanding of analysts' work with these kind of patients. He considered adolescence to be a state of mind that did not depend at all on chronological age. Instead, he described puberty as the collapse of latent structures, once upheld by a severe and obsessive splitting of the self and of objects. According to Meltzer, latency is a sort of waiting, not a mere stage of

DOI: 10.4324/9781003380283-4

development; it is a constellation of defence mechanisms that the child resorts to in order to somehow set aside intense oedipal impulses, to go into the world outside of their family, socialize, and learn, too.

Unconscious defences, by the way, are mostly obsessive mechanisms which, from the Kleinian point of view, are mainly based on an omnipotent control over objects, as well as on the separation of parental objects to avoid coitus, which could result in more babies.

The adolescent's entry into the outside world leads to an increased thirst for knowledge and a desire to acquire new skills, which may be encouraged by parents exerting pressure on them regarding school success, and thus forcing them into a very conflictive situation. This is also the case when it comes to educational institutions, which are in turn under the strain of a "success"-focused society, a topic that is highly debatable in today's world. It is hard to understand what this much-talked-about "success" is all about.

Child and adolescent analysts should rid themselves of any goals or aspirations set for their young patients other than to help them decrease their suffering or alleviate their symptoms. We must not forget that society exerts pressure on psychoanalysts to force us to meet its expectations of setting young people on the road to accomplishment.

Furthermore, the person who had been a child up to that moment believed that their parents knew everything about them, but now, they have abandoned that belief and go in search of a different kind of support – peer support. By means of projective identification, they locate parts of the self onto the different characters of their group of friends: the shy one, the geek, or the athlete, for example. In this way, the internal world is externalized onto a group life, which contributes to reducing the anxiety the adolescent is enduring. Only young persons with the required mental resources achieve this; others lag behind and are left locked inside the world of the "child in the family."

There have been very interesting discussions about whether puberty is thought of as the end of childhood or the beginning of the adolescent process, as Bion stated above. Discussions have also been held about whether it constitutes a stage in and of itself, a space-time of transition from childhood to adulthood, or the passage from endogamy to exogamy.

In my opinion, there is a clear eye within this sort of tornado: a sexed body suddenly bursts in and imposes an enormous psychic workload on the pubescent mind, at a moment when it does not yet have enough elements to process all these changes. And it is not a singular erogenous body: it is a sexed body as long as it is thought of in relation to another.

Like any process of subjectivation, these events must be regarded in their relation to the context of the times they take place in. The pubescent sexed body is defined in its relationship with another body that grants it the status of sexed body. Here the external perspective, from both parents and peers, is of great importance.

With the fall of the latent structure, the typical confusion of the pre-oedipal stage re-emerges (good/bad, feminine/masculine, child/adult), as well as that of erogenous zones. Therefore, total confusion reigns and the young person needs to be contained by their environment in order to process the emotions that drive them to action.

Meltzer (1993) highlights the importance of a peer group at this stage. It is not just about the process of socialization; the peer group serves fundamentally to contain the confusion brought about by projective identification, through which parts of the self are put into play with such force and violence that they inevitably lead to action, something very much characteristic of the behaviour of young people. The core idea is that groups of pubescents/adolescents create a space in which human relationships can be experienced, specifically in the external world, where there are no adults involved.

Whenever we engage in analysis with an adolescent, it is key for us to understand that it is a difficult time for the young person to be interested in exploring their inner world, and that, as a matter of fact, us analysts make part of the adult world that they are constantly defying.

Puberty and its drifts

The changing times of puberty/adolescence have been referenced in the foregoing section. The irruption of the novelty of a sexed body occurs at a time when the young person feels a disturbing discomfort in their way of inhabiting childhood, since they do not have the necessary psychic tools to cope with such a change. They do not own the keys to the adult world either, and everything takes place in a very particular moment in time that Castoriadis (1975) refers to as a time of *alteration*.

I will tackle the issue of time further in the chapter; here I believe it is worthwhile exploring Castoriadis's proposal which is that the rationalist-determinist project established after Plato is fallacious because it does not account for otherness, for the emergence of what is new, for creation, both in terms of individual and collective imagination. It is the appearance of novelty that should be centre-stage; new elements that may be underpinned by what was already existent, but which cannot be inferred therefrom.

There is no way for the world to be a cyclical repetition, nor any proof of a total or fundamental causality. There is no scheme of any succession of events. Castoriadis emphasises approaching the problem of time as *alterity/alteration*, as the emergence of the Other, which gives rise to diverse ways of thinking and being "others." Time, for Castoriadis, implies rupture, emergence, a source of novelty; something that is essentially indeterminate and essentially capable of new determinations; an irruption that occurs as an *incessant self-alteration*.

Puberty is constituted in a conflicting coexistence of the inertia of the broken latent configuration and a truth – arising from drive and from a pushing force – that is persistently demanding to be included. The effort involved in this process is fundamental, and in arriving at the other side, one may be faced with the fact that a space of one's own is yet to be found.

Moreno (2014) puts forward a very interesting and useful idea for analytic practice with pubescents and adolescents. He proposes three potential paths starting off at the pubertal crossroads: event, catastrophe and halt.

In line with Badiou (1988), the *event* points to a radical change that cannot be tied to any preceding circumstance. If the pubescent goes through the adolescent process in a regulated manner, they may develop into a neurotic adult. This cannot always be traced back to the adolescent stage, but it can be inferred that the disturbing novelty, that sort of disruption that has taken place, was eventually processed during the adolescent period and will follow its course into adult life.

The second possible path following the pubertal crisis is *catastrophe*: it occurs when that insistent and disturbing new element is not lodged or inscribed in the person. The overwhelming force of novelty manages to destroy the supports that remained of the structures built with obsessive mechanisms of latency. There are attempts to produce delusional elements and the doors to psychosis are opened – let us not forget that the onset of schizophrenia usually takes place at this stage of life.

It should be underscored that all these processes require containment from the adolescent's environment – both family and society – which should offer space for the processes to unfurl without giving way to severe mental illness. With regard to this topic, Winnicott introduced a strikingly relevant idea in his chapter on adolescence in *Playing and Reality* (Winnicott, 1971). He speaks of "parental abdication", a situation in which parents deliberately delegate responsibility to their children and leave them to deal with all the hostility of adolescence on their own. Hence the increasing clinical occurrences of self-harm, such as the cutting syndrome or eating disorders, which can even come to suicide. I have discussed this topic in detail in a chapter of *Playing and Reality Revisited* (Ungar, 2015).

Resuming Moreno's proposition, the third possible way out of the pubertal crisis is the *halt* of the adolescent process when it fails to produce something radically new. Infantile, latent features remain and can take on pseudoadolescent forms, but the pubescent is stuck in the infantile world, that is, "the world of the child in the family" (Meltzer, 1993).

It is very important to be able to recognize this situation. Not only does it leave the young person inhabiting an infantile universe, but it also may amount to what Meltzer described as "pseudo-maturity". This clinical manifestation carries an important meta-psychological significance, since it is an attempt to bypass the oedipal conflict, which implies a risky proximity to psychosis.

Later on, generally in middle age, a crisis may lead to the catastrophe described above. In such a case, the subject will lack the necessary plasticity to attain a psychic change.

Puberty – adolescence – culture

Since puberty is the beginning of adolescence, it consists of a paradigm in which body, psyche and society are bound together. Historically, culture has provided rites of passage to accompany moments of significant change in a lifetime, like birth, death and marriage. In ancient times, as in some tribal societies today, there were rites of passage from childhood to adulthood.

However, contemporary society does not offer institutionalized rites of passage. Young people have to create their own, so as to become part of the adolescent community; and today's rituals are more akin to tests of courage, as in fairy tales. These may consist of kissing or having sex with someone they have only just met, drinking alcohol to the point of losing consciousness, smoking marijuana or taking other substances, among others.

In our present culture, adolescence has been enshrined as an ideal of longing: children today dream of becoming adolescents as soon as possible, while adults would give anything to be adolescents again. This phenomenon has been closely studied by marketing experts who specially target the adolescent population.

While adolescence seems to have been almost non-existent in medieval times, today it definitely spans a much longer period of time. The fact that young people are the main target of today's marketing agents is evidence of the strong socioeconomic pressure exerted on them to prolong their adolescence. According to statistics, the percentage of people in their late thirties who continue to live with their parents is on the rise; this is added to other characteristics anomalous to chronological age, such as dressing similarly to adolescents, watching TV shows for children (like cartoons), playing video games, collecting superhero magazines and even decorating their bedrooms with dolls or action figures from whatever TV series is "in" at the time.

All of this refers to culture, and since there is no longer any doubt that processes of subjectivation require interaction with the environment, I will now focus on the world we are currently living in and the challenges pubescent children encounter when approaching adulthood.

Admittedly, young people today are lonelier than ever before; no doubt, one of the main reasons for this is the fast pace of modern life and the pressure to succeed. In addition to having adults spending lots of time trying to achieve that success, current times hijack their spaces for playing, both in terms of time and libido that could be shared with children. The latter also tend to have full schedules because, from a very early age, they are steered towards the promised excellence.

Moreover, it has been over three years since the sudden and unexpected outburst of a highly contagious virus with hitherto unknown effects on human health, COVID-19, which swiftly crossed borders and evolved into a pandemic. This humanitarian tragedy shed light on the failure of the prevailing economic system worldwide. Inequities, inequalities in terms of access to education and health, xenophobia, racism, and violence against women and children have become more evident.

Furthermore, in February 2022, a conflict between Ukraine and Russia escalated to a full-scale war and left us perplexed and glued to TV screens and news portals, where we saw images that account for the horror of human destructiveness. This is not a new scenario, but quite the opposite: it evokes in all generations a sad memory, and reminds us that there is a component of human nature that endures and remains – our capacity to destroy our fellow humans as well as Mother Earth. It is also true that, in recent years, we have had to learn to live with uncertainty. Although we have always done so, our powerful defence mechanisms enabled us to deny uncertainty along with our own fragility.

The notion of time

The notion of time we used to grapple with in our daily lives and in our clinical practice has undergone some changes. We were very much used to thinking in terms of continuity, processes, development, evolution. But since the beginning of 2020, we are experiencing a reality that came about suddenly, the main feature of which is disruption. The impact of uncertain and disruptive elements on mental health has been enormous and we cannot yet assess to what extent.

The notions of permanence and certainty (even when these are always relative) have been torn apart. Janine Puget has been working on this topic for several years now, and suggests very firmly in her book that we "raise uncertainty to the category of regulatory principle: it is foreseeable that the unforeseeable will happen" (Puget, 2018). Thus, "the principle of uncertainty establishes a difference between uncertainty as a colloquial term and its place in theory." In psychoanalytic practice, this principle connects us with our fragility and the fragility of our bonds, with the ephemeral and illusory nature of our firm beliefs, and with our notion of ownership over material things.

The COVID-19 pandemic entailed a forced coexistence with uncertainty, plus a rupture of the notion of continuity, which in turn encompasses a relationship between time and movement. The rupture in our experience of time is linked to the concept of *Chronos* – which implies both the circular time of Ancient Greece and Rome and the linear time of Christianity – according to which there is a before and an after, and the basis of which is the origin, that is, the beginning, which may be the creation of the universe or the birth of Christ. The discontinuity we are experiencing also deeply affects the ideal of progress of the Modern Era, fragmenting our possibility of making plans and predicting any portion of the future with some sort of certainty.

The pandemic brought about an additional painful reality: children were quick to understand that they could be the vectors of infection, and thus realized at a very early age that they had to take care of their elders, while fearing that they could be blamed for their death, an intolerable responsibility at such a young age. As such, we saw an increase in clinical manifestations of anxiety crises, sleep disorders, eating disorders, and acute phobias in children and adolescents, as well as a refusal to leave home.

Another way of referring to time that has appeared in many publications in the last three years is a quote by from *Hamlet*: "The time is out of joint." This quote had previously been employed by thinkers such as Deleuze and Derrida, among others, and has been used often because it fits the description of a traumatic experience, of a genuine disruption in the face of the threat of a virus that caused fear of contagion and death, isolation and deprivation of personal contact, confinement and a subsequent immobility.

Our times have also been referred to as *dystopian*. The term "dystopia" points to the fictional representation of a future society with undesirable characteristics. One of the best-known dystopian societies was the one created by George Orwell in his novel *Nineteen Eighty-Four* (1949). Dystopia is a subgenre of science fiction literature that has become very popular among adolescents. It is considered to be the opposite to the term "utopia," which refers to a fantasy, an ideal society that seems perfect but is impossible. A utopia is almost a dream, something we long for but which does not really exist.

We are living a painful reality: first, the COVID-19 pandemic, the war in Ukraine and an increasingly threatening climate tragedy. The war persists and is further proof that everything is constantly changing and that possible projects are subject to disruptions. The world is on edge and the dreaded effects of worldwide conflicts are already taking place. In addition to casualties, there is an increase in the rate of displacement, with thousands of people fleeing and seeking asylum in countries near or far away from home. Uprootedness, xenophobia and their consequences on the processes of subjectivation are plain to see. Those of us who work in psychoanalysis with children and adolescents must be present and offer all the possibilities of our discipline to also intervene in environments other than our offices and institutions.

The clinical, technical and theoretical foundations of psychoanalysis can only grow and expand if we pay attention to and engage with the problems of the world we inhabit. It is the difficulties in our practice, or rather the obstacles that our clinical work faces us with, that lead us to question the theory, which then usually translates into new hypotheses. Obstacles compel us to leave the comfort zone of the theories that are at the core of the model of the mind each of us works with; they force us to stop and think, and in doing so, they lead us to try and effect changes.

What we are going through following the pandemic is a clear example of this: it is an obstacle that brought the world to a halt and forced us to make changes at every step. Now, we work and teach online using our digital devices, and we even organize our scientific events this way. Undoubtedly, today's approach to psychoanalysis is completely different from when this discipline was born. As analysts we know that in order for the transference to happen, the analytical setting is *sine qua non*. I am not referring to the formal conditions of the setting, but to a notion – of a more psychoanalytic nature, in my opinion – that is to be internalised and is linked to the so-called *analytic attitude.*

The setting is the technical aspect of the analytical method. The method is also what we offer to our patients, and according to Freud's definition, research and therapy converge in it. In the case of children and adolescents, more than any other age group, the setting must be malleable to accommodate their different modes of communication.

Another major topic of discussion in psychoanalysis is the so-called "fading or fall of the paternal function". As we all know, ever since Freud's crucial approach, the topic of the father is tied to the Oedipus complex. I have always wondered about the legitimacy of separating or isolating the three oedipal actors (father, mother, child), who are inextricably linked within the complex approach, forming a basic structure.

The paternal role does not come about suddenly; it does not come by inheritance – not even as an ancestral heritage. It is a sort of daily and prolonged weaving of the bond with the child that results in the man becoming a father. This has little to do with the concrete caring for the baby since birth, but with a slow and silent reformulation of the parenting function at each step of the way, which is tested while simultaneously devised and exercised. That is why I prefer to use the term *parentality*, which seems to me to cover the surface where two circles overlap and create a shared territory: those circles would be becoming a mother and becoming a father.

Today's model of the family is far removed from the modern ideal of the family that prevailed at the outset of psychoanalysis. The children and adolescents who come to our practice may be members of other family configurations, such as blended families, single-parent families, same-sex couples, etc.

Furthermore, a very interesting topic arises in the field of filiation as a result of technological developments that question what previously seemed irreducible: biological paternity. At this point in time, we no longer mistake – or should not mistake – the paternal function for the role played by a man who is called "father" and lives with a family in which he is the father of the children and the husband of the wife. Nowadays it is not necessary for a man to fulfil this role and be a father at the same time. This function may be performed by someone else, who does not necessarily have to be male. This is why I find it appropriate to speak of a weakening of the paternal function, an attenuation, or *affaiblissement,* as French authors put it. The resulting effect can be sensed in some of the manifestations of current pathologies in childhood and adolescence.

Another issue to be considered is the fact that the traditional support platform for the transition from childhood to adolescence – the family and, secondly, educational institutions – is currently sharing protagonism with the digital world.

Children and adolescents spend much of their time on social media, ever more so in the last two years. Group exchanges are not necessarily happening at the school playground during recess anymore, nor at the club, or any specific geographical area. Now, the meeting place is predominantly virtual. The territory for encounters lies in smartphones that are constantly updated with more and more features.

A further topical issue is the penetration of the dialect used on social media into everyday language. It is the media that determine whether someone exists or not. This can help us understand why it is so important for an adolescent that their "existence" be corroborated by a commented post and an acceptable number of followers on social media.

Numerous questions arise: How is subjectivation produced and sociability constructed in a context such as the current one, which is strongly mediatised, where there is a preponderance of image, exposure and visibility, and in which celebrity is exalted by mass media? How does one create and preserve the intimate space that is essential for the analysis to unfold? What has all this time of uncertainty and isolation taught us?

Even before the pandemic, we were no longer alone with our patients, as the setting also began to accept late arrival notices or requests for schedule changes via text messages, or patients show us something "very important" on YouTube or a "life-changing" chat conversation with their ex-partner.

So far, I have made reference to changes in practice. I am convinced that changes in theory are starting to become evident, giving that, as historians say, history cannot be written while it is happening – a certain distance is required to observe the changes, to describe them and to reflect upon them. My impression is that the mental mechanisms used by children and adolescents are closer to splitting than to repression. I do think repression is used as well, but young peoples' simultaneous interactions through social media – for example, watching television, chatting, watching a YouTube video or sending a WhatsApp message on their phone – are more understandable to me if I consider them a splitting and dissociation of various levels of the self that allows them to scatter, or conversely focus, their attention on several things at once.

In conclusion, I reiterate the idea that changes will become much more evident in hindsight. Still, we must show openness to them; not from an adolescent-like stance, but from a position of genuine wonder and desire to learn.

References

Badiou, A. (1988). *Being and Event*. New York: Continuum.

Bion, W.R. (1977). Emotional Turbulence. In: P. Hartocollis (ed.), *Borderline Personality Disorders: The Concept, the Syndrome, the Patient*. New York: International Universities Press, p. 3.

Castoriadis, C. (1975). *The Imaginary Institution of Society*. Cambridge, MA: MIT Press.

Meltzer, D. & M. Harris (1993). *Adolescence. Talks and Papers by Donald Meltzer and Martha Harris*, ed. M. Harris Williams. The Meltzer Harris Trust.

Moreno, J. (2014). *La infancia y sus bordes* [Childhood and its Borders]. Buenos Aires: Paidós.

Orwell, G. (1949). *Nineteen Eighty-Four*, London: Secker and Warburg.

Puget, J. (2018). *Subjetivación discontinua y Psicoanálisis. Incertidumbres y certezas* [Discontinuous Subjectivation and Psychoanalysis. Uncertainties and Certainties]. Buenos Aires: Lugar Editorial.

Ungar, V. (2015). Playing and Reality Revisited: Clinical Practice with Adolescents in the Twenty-First Century. In: Saragnano, G. & Seulin, C. (eds), *Playing and Reality Revisited. A New Look at Winnicott's Classic Work*. London: Routledge.

Winnicott, D.W. (1971) *Playing and Reality*. London: Routledge.

5   What prevents adolescents from suicide?[1]

François Ladame

We usually approach the issue of suicide in adolescence through the investigation of factors we know are promoting the enactment of suicidal ideas. These factors may relate to psychopathology, clinical symptoms and/or the socio-cultural environment (including the family).

I have written many books and papers on suicide in adolescence (Ladame, 1981, Ladame, Ottino & Pawlak, 1995, Ladame 2008). They all follow this line. Today, my reflections will go exactly the opposite way. I propose not to ask the question: *what drives an adolescent to suicide?* but instead, *what may prevent an adolescent to kill himself?* A more provocative version would be: *why all adolescents don't kill themselves?* To put the question in psychoanalytical words, I will ask about the kind of changes which must take place in the adolescent psyche in order later on in his life to function as a safeguard against suicide. I stress "safeguard" because I believe not only in the complexity of the psychic apparatus but also in its deep heterogeneity. This implies that we have to work with mere indices of what is going on in the different layers of the psyche and we are not allowed to assume that a catastrophe like suicide will never happen.

One of the developmental tasks of adolescence is to "own" his/her own life. The ownership of one's own life means feeling responsible for it, taking care of it and value it notwithstanding the reality that one has not been self-engendered. My assumption is that an adolescent can only get there once he has been able first to regard suicide as possible, then to identify with the caring and protective side of the objects of his past.

"I am a living 'subject' but I have the power, should I decide it, to end my life." Let's try to unfold this very condensed statement. To be able to feel myself a "subject", or an "I", I must first have accomplished three fundamental tasks: 1) become the owner of my body, 2) of my drives, and 3) of my thoughts. The construction of the "subject" – a favourite concept of the French psychoanalysts – is synonymous for me with building up one's own identity (Ladame, 2003). It is the step that allows entering adulthood with a basal security, protected from agonizing or traumatic anxieties. The ownership of the body means the ownership of the mature sexual body, either male or female, while giving up the illusory fantasy of a body which might be both male and female or neither one nor the other. It also means that there is no

DOI: 10.4324/9781003380283-5

longer any "code share" with the parents, as it happened during childhood, when they were still more or less responsible for the good state and health of the child's body. Finally, it means the mourning of the illusion of having once possessed the body of the oedipal parent (I stress "illusion" because the child never possessed it; at most, in a very remote past, he has been in a somehow undifferentiated relationship with the body of the pre-oedipal mother.) But I will return later to this point because it is especially relevant to this discussion.

Let us consider, then, the issue of the ownership of one's own drives. Unlike very young adolescents, the older ones can no longer blame others for their drives and moreover the action of their drives. They must now take full responsibility for them. The positive aspect of becoming the owner of one's drives is the possibility of completing the identity's construction of an adult male or female when internalization supersedes projective mechanisms. *"My sexuality is mine, my sexual desires are mine"*, and the same is true for the aggressiveness, and it is my freedom to make use of them in consistence with an evolved superego. Should the adolescent still hold others responsible for his drives, the subject, the self, would be deprived from one's own energy, one's own fuel, if I dare say so. The negative side of the story is the accountability towards one's conscience, one's superego. To withstand it, feelings of guilt must not be overwhelming; otherwise, regression may override progression. In order to escape either such a counter-evolution or a developmental deadlock, the attacks against the internalized parents must not persist with the belief that the action of the drives resulted in their destruction. In other words, the adolescent must not be trapped in the conviction that he/she succeeded in destroying the oedipal couple; should it be the case, the outcome would be either an impasse in the identification process, leaving a gap in the construction of the subject, or an identification with dead objects (melancholic identification). Moreover, the adolescent has to disengage from the *primal scene* and accept himself as a third party, that is, free from the relationship between the parental imagos. His ability to stand alone relies on the strength of the narcissistic grounds.

Regarding drives, there is another very important point I would like to stress. The safeguard against a drive outburst resulting in a destructive act relies on their *binding*. The free instinct – destructive or death instinct – has to be constantly bound, giving rise to greater "units" – sexual or life instinct – as well as to psychic representations (which may be unconscious, preconscious and/or conscious). Daydreaming, the ability to build pictures in one's mind, relies on such a binding process where the activity of the Preconscious plays a central role. At the border between an undifferentiated instinctual outburst resulting in a violent act and a "controlled" action, the capacity of daydreaming or fantasying is a major safeguard.

Let us now consider the issue of the ownership of one's own thoughts, which is especially relevant in today's context. On the one hand, it implies the child's capacity to go beyond the feeling that his parents "know" what he is thinking, that they know whether he is lying or not; it means the progression from the feeling that the parents have the power to "read" inside his/her mind towards the security to be the owner – the only owner – of the content of the thinking apparatus. In other words, if one's body might be raped, it is in no way true for the thought. On the other hand, this development includes the newly acquired capacity of the adolescent to take oneself as an object of reflection. We may say that a "subject" must be there – a subject has to be constructed – to open to the possibility to see oneself as an object (an object of thinking). The door is now open for the adolescent to reflect not only on the issue of life and death but above all *his* life and *his* death, the origin of his own life and consideration of suicide as a possibility.

Even if many adolescents try to convince themselves, whatever the price they pay, that they are self-engendered, none of us has ever been at the origin of one's own life. Hence the haunting question of the debt towards one's genitors. A patient of mine put it very clearly when she asked the question: "*What does it mean to be indebted to someone for my own life?*" What does it mean and, moreover, what does it imply? You have probably guessed that the patient I am alluding to has been, for years and years, a rebel, revolting against the order of the world that assigns a place to each human being and conducts succession of the generations. Her rebellion drove her to endanger her life to the point that she might have died.

The adolescent and future adult must survive the reality that he is not self-engendered, and he does not owe his parents his own life. To be able to narcissistically survive such a reality without either falling apart or feeling bound to remain in a state of childish dependency, the narcissism must have been sufficiently strengthened to offer the security of possessing an identity on one's own right and having successfully identified with a *living* couple of parents. Through this identification with a couple of living and creative parents, the adolescent is also freed of the burden of a supposed eternal debt.

But we are far from the end of the story! The construction of the adult identity, of the "I", of a "subject" who exists on one's own right implies a *process of differentiation* (Ladame, 2003). This process undoubtedly began in the early years of life, but its completion is the hallmark along the route from adolescence to adulthood. It implies different levels: fundamentally, at a subjective level the differentiation between subject – self – and object, but also the difference between male and female which is fully different from the one between boy and girl acknowledged early in childhood. Sexes are complementary, both are "castrated", and each of them needs the other one in order to temporarily feel complete. This new acknowledgment should go along with the differentiation between *needs*, which may involve survival, and *desires*, whose frustration no more imply the being, the essence of the subject. If the two levels are undifferentiated or regressively confused, the frustration felt when a desire is not satisfied may give rise to such a narcissistic hurt that the narcissism is threatened to collapse, leaving "murder" as the only way out. And unfortunately, the killing of the object implies the killing of the self because the object is an internal one, and is not differentiated from the self.

The differentiation process I am speaking of also concerns the differences between generations and between life and death with the irreversibility of the latter. This notion is supposedly acquired in middle adolescence, but we should be cautious about it. Suicide is not an intellectual act but an emotional one. And we all know from our work with patients in grief how fast a regressive stand comes along with the intensity of the sorrow and may give rise either to the belief that the deceased and beloved one will return or to false perceptions of his/her presence. Therefore, I would certainly not consider cognitive or intellectual achievements as a safeguard against the risk of suicide. As you may have understood, I shall mainly trust the firmness of the narcissistic grounds and feel concerned by any indices of a current narcissistic fragility.

***

It may unfortunately happen that an adolescent finds himself trapped into a paradoxical situation regarding the issue of life and death and the demand to find a way out the primal scene. I shall try to illustrate the complexity of such situations by letting a patient speak.

Henri was close to 15 years when I met him in the particular setting of *individual psychoanalytic psychodrama.* With the exception of those working or trained in French speaking countries, clinicians are usually not very familiar with this setting. Therefore I will briefly explain it so that you may understand how my colleagues and I were able to grasp a great deal of information about Henri's psychic functioning during only a few sessions (see Ladame & Catipovic, 1998).

Maybe one of the easiest ways to figure out what psychoanalytic psychodrama looks like is to recall Hamlet calling in a troupe of wandering players to bring out the truth – a truth as yet unknown but nevertheless already known. Shakespeare was not content merely to lend materiality to his hero's conscience, which haunted him in the form of the ghost, but constructed a play within the play, a stage within the stage, to enable him to think the unthinkable. That is, in short, what psychodrama is about.

Three fundamental rules underlie psychodrama: 1) putting forward and organising a scene with the help of the play director; 2) playing (with six to eight male and female co-therapists); 3) make-believe while playing. The approach of psychodrama proceeds in the opposite direction of that of classical analytic therapies: it begins with action (playing) and continues by thinking what has been played and arousing conscious and unconscious fantasies.

The setting itself, including as it does the presence of the group of co-therapists, constitutes a reassuring containing device. The playing in psychodrama involves not a patient alone but one interacting with the co-therapists. Owing to the availability of those several co-therapists, the psychodrama play technique offers the patient a plural or conflictualized view of one and the same psychic "event" in situations where the conflict is unthinkable and its contradictory aspects either cause confusion or else are evacuated. But the greatest value of psychodrama is that it affords a configuration from which the third person can at no time be "excluded". Patients relate successively to a director with whom they speak but don't play, watched by the co-therapists, and to the group of co-therapists, with whom they play, watched by the director, on whom they know they can call if necessary.

Henri had been treated with individual psychotherapy for nearly one year when his psychotherapist requested the help of psychodrama because he felt the two were in an impasse and he was unable to tackle the patient's affects as well as his relationship with his father. Henri was in agreement with the procedure and gave permission to his therapist to disclose to our team information about his life before any decision whether we would welcome him or not for a few exploratory sessions.

Henri is HIV positive. He was infected by her mother during pregnancy, and the mother had been contaminated by her partner, Henri's father. The contamination was discovered very late, close to the term of the pregnancy. Mother and son were put on HAART (highly active anti-retroviral therapy). Henri is still on treatment, whereas his mother had in the meantime divorced and, with her new partner, was able a few years ago to give birth to an unhurt little girl (that means that virus in her blood, if any, is not detectable). Besides HAART, Henri also received injections of growth hormone for growth retardation. Our group was quite surprised that Henri gave permission to disclose so many intimate details to strangers, to people he hadn't yet met with. During our preliminary discussion with the psychotherapist, it became obvious that so doing he sent us a message about the danger he thought he potentially represented for all of us. In other words, the disclosure had to do with the patient's aggression and his anxiety of losing control on his destructive drives.

At the very beginning of the first session, when sitting with the play director, Henri insists on reading a story he has just written on his laptop and printed before coming and seeing us. The story is about George and Gallagher. *George is travelling through India after running away from his home where he was beaten by his parents and he meets a friend, Gallagher. The two of them go together for a walk. They are soon followed by two-armed people in black dress and hoods. Unlike George, Gallagher notices them in time and is able to hide himself. George is shot to death. He was the only friend Gallagher had ever had!* And Henri adds: *Anytime Gallagher feels close to someone else; the latter dies.* I leave you imagine how our whole psychodrama team felt while listening to Henri and how much we all had to struggle with ourselves in order to contain the amount of affects while remaining available and therapeutically active for the patient. The play director asks Henri whether or not he wants to play the scene as he described it or make changes. He answers yes and distributes the roles. He chooses to play George and gives the role of Gallagher to one of the male co-therapists. For the second scene, Henri suggests playing something he has lived out a few days ago during an excursion with schoolmates at the lakeside. The small group of adolescents were seemingly offended and threatened by two rowers. To start with Henri stresses how scared he felt; however, while playing the scene it occurs that he has himself thrown stones at the boat before the rowers reacted so strongly.

I might go into further details about the progress of the sessions. However, I'll limit myself to highlight our deductions from the scenes played by the patient. Henri presented us with a deadly primal scene he has locked in while undifferentiated parents (the two-armed people in black dress and hood) shoot one's load – a fatal discharge.[2] Hence the paradox – not to mention the aporia – Henri is faced with:

1   The sexual relationship of the parents was carrier of death and has given birth to a child (Henri) who feels himself also to be a death carrier (hence the supposed dangerousness I alluded to above).
2   Should the parents' relationship have been credited with love, Henri would not have been born; they would have made love with a condom!

In that way, Henri's case is a tragic example of an extreme "tensioning", up to a paradox, of the issue of life and death as it presents in adolescence.

How might it happen that Henri becomes the owner of his own life? That he becomes able to invest his life with a positive value and take care of it? That he internalizes a life carrying primal scene? We'll know that only in the future. What we currently know is that this adolescent is locked up between the solutions of either identifying with a dangerous, death-carrier parent or non-being, the issue of negative narcissism. The first solution would mean becoming a "killer" himself, an identification conflicting with both the superego demands and the ego ideal aims. As Henri is entering middle adolescence, he is more and more preoccupied with dating and sexual relations with girl-friends; therefore, the conflict is exacerbated. Alternatively, instead of being a killer, he might either become a "self-killer" or feel attracted towards negativity, non-being and nothingness. Therefore, you may not be surprised to learn that Henri became so suicidal that he needed in-patient care for a few weeks.

Let us now come back to the central point of my presentation: as the issue of life and death is in the heart of adolescent development, it makes sense to ask, "why all adolescents don't kill themselves?". The issue of life and death is inescapable, and everyone has to find an answer to while building up one's own identity. In my view, it is not possible to invest one's life, to give it a *positive* value without having first envisaged the possibility of ending it. I am weighing my words carefully because I am far from being an apologist of suicide in adolescence. What I want to stress is that the capability to regard suicide as possible goes hand in hand with the opening of a space for thinking where the subject can take oneself as an object of reflection. In that sense it contributes in a decisive way to the achievement of the identity's construction: *I am all the more able to "own" my life – and disengage from the narcissistic aporia that I was not at its founding – that I have contemplated the possibility to bring it to an end.* [3]

This space for thinking becomes the container of all the daydreams and fantasies where one can imagine oneself as dead and imagine the tearful others present at one's funeral. At that moment, my temporarily defeated narcissism is invigorated, fully revived. The loss of self-esteem and the risk of dropping into a negative narcissism are hopefully over. *If so, many people are crying over me, they must be fond of me; and if so many people love me, I may be allowed to love me as well.* At that moment in the sequence of the thinking process, the enactment of the suicidal fantasy is no more compulsory because the thought has fully achieved its function of trial action (Freud, 1933).

What I just described is for me one of the main safeguards against the risk of suicide. And it is an achievement of adolescence. I now want to emphasize another major safeguard I hinted at as I spoke of the ownership of the body. It will take us back from adolescence to the very early development because this shelter has to do with the primal relationship between the infant's body and the body of his/her mother.[4]

Eglé Laufer developed the idea of *the body as an internal object*. This notion allows conceptualizing the memory traces of the *emotional experience* of the relation between the infant body and his mother as well as his relationship with the maternal body. In that way this notion, while focusing on the affective dimension of the experience, is different from the concept of body image which is built up from the sensory experiences and perceptions. Most important, this "internal object" is not only constituted by the memory traces of the infant's pleasant or painful experiences in relation with his mother's body but also of the traces of the pleasure or displeasure felt by the mother in relation with her baby's body. Eglé Laufer gives credit to Winnicott's aphorism "a baby doesn't exist without a mother", but she also acknowledges that a mother exists from the beginning: the mother is at the same time consubstantial and separated. Therefore, only those traces which may be shared in a *mutually rewarding* way can be introjected and form this "loved" internal object that is narcissistically invested.

In some ways, the concept developed by Eglé Laufer may be seen as close to the French notion of "corps érotique" (erotic body), but it is much more elaborated and less ambiguous avoiding any confusion between surface and depth. The body as internal object containing the fantasy of a "complete" and omnipotent body while united with the mother's body serves as a major defence – not to say the only defence – against helplessness and traumatic anxieties. It also forms a kind of narcissistic "shield" one can rely on while growing up in order to feel secure and pleased with one's own body. It is probably the best protection against a destructive hatred of one's body, hence against suicide, because we should not forget that suicide always implies the "murder" of one's own hated body.

At the opposite, the infant who was not able to feel sufficiently secure and loved in his primal experience of narcissistic union with the mother's body is forced to build up an idealized body image when he has to face the reality of separateness and differentiation at the oedipal level. This idealized image permits to maintain a fantasy of omnipotent fusion. At least until puberty when the reality of the transformation of one's own body gives the final kick to that fantasy. The confrontation with the mother's "sexual" body mirroring the adolescent's mature body leaves room for a hatred of the sexually potent male or female body as being responsible for the illusion of narcissistic union having been swept away.

Now comes the question hiding behind all these theoretical remarks: what can we do with an adolescent or adult patient who was not able to form a loved, erotic, internal object during early childhood? According to my experience, only the analytic setting offers the possibility to regress to these archaic levels of development; to such a level of regression where it is possible, for both analysed and analyst, to revisit the primitive bodily experiences. But how many of all our young patients are or will ever be in analysis? This means that inevitably some patients will die by suicide.

I have been treating severely ill adolescents for more than 40 years. You may understand that, over the years, it unfortunately happened that a few of them either irreversibly destroyed, in one way or another, their mature sexual body or died by suicide. One way I have found to cope with these tragic outcomes, with these failures – mine and theirs – was to condense theory and experience through another way of expressing myself. Some years ago, I wrote a text, a poem, which came back to my mind while writing this chapter. Its title is "Identity in Questions" and I am grateful to Sue Rose who is both translator and poet for the quality of her translation from French into English.

It will be my way to conclude, with the hope that words will speak for themselves.

You were 18 years old at least
Identity in questions
François Ladame

Thomas dreams
I leave home, I am attacked

It's hot, it's sweating crowds

I try to escape, I am pursued,
someone is hot on my heels
But I'm running faster and faster

Breakneck descent
Down the Path at the End of the World
Some guy tries to hit me
with a baseball bat

Thomas wakes
Was that Double trouble?
Potential violence
A mixture: West Side
And the side paths of the Bois
Sinister faces, highly strung,
Slip of his tongue,
gallows bird,
Oh, he was well hung at the end.
Dream or nightmare
Sandra
Pushed out of the maternal nest
you took to the streets as a prostitute
living-dead flesh treading the pavements
Cry for help quest for a woman's identity
Destroyed
She was never built up
Destroyed

Why this violence
Doubles
Ecstasy or S&M scene
The glass can turn into a play of mirrors
Psyche, your mirror is my salvation
One last fix Serge and you went and locked
yourself in the shithouse
Why this violence
I is under threat
Where is this threat
The other
The other
I is I hates the pleasure of the other
I is I hates the desire of the other
He knew a bit already, Le Lorrain
learned philosopher about dreams
one hundred years ago
"Without serious fatigue,
Without being obliged to have recourse to that long and stubborn
struggle which
exhausts and wears away pleasures sought."

And you Sébastien
Your brother, your double
one summer evening you found him
at the entrance to the park
in the branches of the chestnut tree

And you became no one
But were you ever I
Yes you were
Yes When you began to
dress in pink
and you wanted to have skin
like peaches and cream
and reverse the order of things
Why this violence
I is powerless
Why this violence
I is more power
Doubles
Don Juan and Leporello

Oscar and Alfred Siss and Unn
A blaze locked inside melting ice
The Ice Palace will fall apart
In the spring in the stream it will sink
and in its crash it will sweep Unn away
Doubles

You will not all be lucky enough to become
Mozart or Chéreau
or Tarjei Vesaas

Why this violence

"C o n s u b s t a n t a t i o"
"C o n s u b s t a n t I a l I s"
Hallelujah
What You said inseparable
You must be kidding You really took me in with your illusion

An illusion
Was it that you were searching for Sinead
your eyes turned towards fresh running water
when you clambered up the garden ladder
and climbed the tall tulip tree
Rebellious rock singer
your red hair could
throw flames
And the lake that evening
became a bronze mirror
And you believed you saw the unknown at last
The unknown which was already running out on you

Notes

1 A shorter version of this chapter was presented at the Brent Centre for Young People, 50th Anniversary Conference, London, 27–28 October 2017.
2 Here I am facing a linguistic problem I was only able to solve approximately. In French, we use the expression "tirer un coup" both for "fucking" and "shooting". In other words, Henri's imaginary story beautifully illustrates how he is at the same time fascinated and trapped in a violent primal scene from he is not yet able to extricate himself.
3 As we all know, when this aporia is leading the psychic functioning, it becomes a powerful suicide promoting factor with the following formula: as I could not decide on my birth I still can decide on my death (as I was not the alpha, I still can be the omega).
4 I am indebted to my close, and alas, late friend Eglé Laufer as the first psychoanalyst who really tried to elaborate this issue (cf. E. Laufer, 2005, Le corps comme objet interne, *Adolescence* 23(2): 363–379).

References

Freud, S. (1933) *New Introductory Lectures on Psychoanalysis. S.E.* XXIII. London: Hogarth Press.

Ladame, F. (1981). *Les tentatives de suicide des adolescents*. Paris: Masson.

Ladame, F., Ottino, J. & Pawlak, C. (eds) (1995). *Adolescence et suicide*. Paris: Masson.

Ladame, F. (2003). *Les éternels adolescents*. Paris: Odile Jacob.

Ladame, F. (2008). Treatment Priorities after Adolescent Suicide Attempts. In: Briggs, S., Lemma, A., & Crouch, W. (eds), *Relating to Self-harm and Suicide: Psychoanalytic Perspectives on Practice, Theory and Research*. London: Routledge, pp. 72–79.

Ladame, F. & Perret-Catipovic, M. (1998). *Jeu, fantasmes et réalités: Le psychodrame psychanalytique à l'adolescence*. Paris: Masson.

Laufer, E. (2005). Le corps comme objet interne. *Adolescence* 23(2): 363–379.

6 Effects of adolescent debut on the infantile super-ego

Carlos Moguillansky

Background

Theories about adolescence have gradually shifted from the conception of a life stage to the notion of a process, and various aspects of clinical practice have conceived of adolescence as a transformation. Freud in *Three Essays on the Theory of Sexuality* (1905) spoke of the metamorphosis of puberty. Peter Blos (1962) pointed out the individuation process, Raymond Cahn (1991, 2016) proposed the work of subjectivation, José Bleger (1971) and Ricardo Avenburg (1973) spoke of family desymbiotization. All these authors found in adolescence a life passage marked by separation, segregation, differentiation and the final integration of young people with their origins. These connected events tend to be conceived as a passage – the life crisis between childhood and adulthood – or as a change in the psychic and anthropological nature of such a metamorphosis. Freud indicated in it the discovery of the sexual object and the constitution of preliminary pleasure, prior to genital pleasure. Another unique event that accompanies these two happenings is the *discovery of the subject*. Young people find a perspective that sets them up as a subject differentiated from others. This is determined by their life and sexual history, but in turn, it decides their present and their future. Philippe Gutton (1996) noted, in a fitting summary: "Adolescence is not reduced to an end of child development, erroneously left aside for a long time, but a debut, indeed, an origin, certainly to an organizational crisis, above all a revolution." The three global regions of psychoanalysis reached the same hypothesis. In adolescence there is a crisis about a legacy. The dialectics between the adolescent's cultural tradition and their personal initiative leads to a dramatic synthesis of its components. The forces present strive to impose their desires and cancel out the obstacles in their way. Thus they re-edit a psychic conflict that leads to a compromise, which Freud postulated as the main evolutionary drive.

The crisis marked by overcoming these conflicting forces, in this kind of dialectic *Aufhebung* (Hegel, 1807),[1] is reflected in transformations in the three psychic instances – the id, the ego, and the super-ego. Here I want to describe the most notable changes that occur in the super-ego, following the work of Edith Jacobson (1954) and Peter Blos (1962). Jacobson described the

DOI: 10.4324/9781003380283-6

passage from the archaic infantile super-ego to the super-ego in keeping with the reality of the current ego. Blos described the pre-pubertal super-ego as an uncastrated giant, similar to the pre-Oedipal phallic mother. His descriptions help define the evolutionary movement, regardless of age, as they are phases in the super-ego metamorphosis towards adulthood. The infantile super-ego is presented as an ethical being, omnipotent and omniscient, offering guarantees in action and protecting the ego from uncertainty. In many cases, it takes on supernatural traits, like a god, or assumes the character of a romantic hero, like an ideal ego or a comic book character. The idealization of the infantile super-ego is parallel to the persecutory character of its tyrannical morality. This drives demanding acts against itself – harm, mutilations and suicide attempts – or against third parties – aggressive assaults – which seek to annihilate the moral pain and, with it, the world of the young person. The violence of these self and hetero aggressive attacks shows the conflictive intensity of the dialogue between the super-ego and the ego.

This conflict turns critical in the debut process, in that it argues the prohibitions and threats of expulsion of the infantile super-ego, as the institution that houses and sustains it is called into crisis. In this case, the super-ego adopts qualities of interdiction or of inter-subjective non-tyrannical agreement, as an ethical rule that emerges from the desire of the young person themself and of those close to them. And institutional prohibition remains a social instance that operates by default every time the post-debut super-ego fails in its function – in the way that justice acts with an antisocial being, when society reassumes its guardian function at the individual's ethical failing. In the mature super-ego two distinct ethics live side by side: one institutional and prohibitive, and the other interdictive. Their apparent similarity of form contrasts with their fundamental differences, as can be seen in the differences between legal truth and ethical truth.

***

The debut detaches the young person from the origin in which they grew and differentiates them from the syncretic tradition that marked them as a child. The young person performs a novel recombination and appropriates their life project around two parallel aspects: a) their affiliation to the institutions that support them – when their desire to belong to an institution identifies them adhesively to the customs of the group, a community or institution and b) their filiation to the ancestors that they recreate from their desire. Their filiation differs from identification, as their desire inverts the direction of the lineage. That change produces disidentifications and reformulations of previous relationships. The young person establishes themself in a centrifugal process that recedes from their current desire towards ancestors that they illuminate as necessary archetypes of their own past – now reconstructed retroactively by their new vision of themself. In short, their metamorphosis appeals to the two poles of the psychic conflict: the unconscious desire and the identifications of the ego. And it generates two opposite lineages: with the family models of their identifications to the current ego, and from the current desire of their adolescent crisis to those past archetypes illuminated by them. In this process, defensive and structuring actions participate in opposite directions, co-existing and cooperating with each other.

This dialectics makes a compromise between the familiar symbiotic component, which blurs the individual, and the young person's differentiating initiative. The young person proposes an act of individuation from a symbiosis – as Blos, Bleger and Avenburg think – or they differentiate themselves in a work of subjectivation – as Cahn thinks. All the positions believe necessary the appearance of a *subject* – an unconscious *who* – who will take responsibility for making decisions in this project. The solution of this conflictive dialectics comes between the syncretic plane of the family and social identificatory legacy and the young person's critical attitude, which gives them a differentiating initiative. Thus originates the *Aufhebung* of the debut, synthetizing the different conflictive elements in a unique dramatic act. As a result, the young person sets up a critical opposition, of enormous critical interest, between an ambiguous element – derived from infantile symbiosis – and a personal version disassociated from ambiguity.

Every adolescent creates two family frames, constructed by two different acts: in their *identification* with family ancestors, they construct their affiliation with the family institution; and in their *filiation*, they organize a symbolic family based on their most original and personal desire, which often contradicts their official family history. The semiosis that emerges from that unlikely framing is a point of evolutionary pause, in which each young person reconstructs, recombines and remodels the lines of their tradition and desire, in an amalgam full of synergies and ruptures, co-operations and conflicts, ambiguities and differentiations. In that recombination, each young person adapts to what is given; they give themselves a new order and appropriate their current and future project.

> I have used the phrase 'adolescent debut' for the effect resulting from that synthesizing recombination, as that act instals a new order and a new state of things, which emerge from the unique sexual position that each young person assumes about their sex, their life and their life role.
>
> (Moguillansky, 2012).

Those planes are synergic with each other. And for the same reason, they also show solidarity in the genesis of the symptoms that emerge in them with a similar format.

***

The adolescent debut includes different expressions, but its central nature lies in being an act, if this defines the essentially human aspect of a decision that transcends the idea of a conduct or behaviour. This act is the most authentic decision of the most intimate and personal *who*. In it, the young person, probably unwittingly, undergoes or marks the turning point of their life. In that decision, they appropriate and assume a personal expressive focus, which is set apart from that of their relatives. That act is observed in Dora, in the young homosexual woman, in the Wolf Man and the Rat Man. Aside from the different expressions of their neurosis, they show the moment when they appropriate and assume their fate as their own.

And although the appropriation of the debut tends to be a distinctive deed of the adolescent crisis, it is also seen in life crises in other moments in life, whenever a discovery, grief or an accident trigger a scene dormant in the characterological institution of their life. The debut is no more than the decision – as expression in an act – of a potency that awaits its moment to be triggered. When it occurs, it is a state of exception with no going back. The examples of Breuer and Freud illustrate the situation. Both experienced the same encounter with hysteria. Breuer faced the tension of sex embodied in Anna O. and retreated from it. Freud, in turn, sustained his position and assumed the risky gesture of his action. A unique certainty accompanied him even in the initial bitterness of a difficult beginning. That encounter changed Freud's life. And its effects can still be noted in us. With more modesty, that same risky act is triggered in all young people and drives them to be who they are. Even if their decision is an act of surrender to another will, as in that case, their surrender is not a simple act of submission, but a personal decision to obey – out of love, guilt, desire or any other reason. At this critical point we see the different and possible actions of the super-ego. It imposes two different ethics: prohibition and interdiction. And these are at the beginning and the end of a critical transformation, which sets up an individual differentiation and a personal attitude about norms. That ethical act is at the centre of the decision of the adolescent debut.

***

In some cases juvenile rebellion presents as a defensive alternative to the pain of the debut. Is this rebellion the obstacle to the symbolic process of breaking? Or does it appear as a substitute defence when the symbolic break does not occur? Rebellion and the debut are not parallel, but rather contrary. The release of parental authority is not the main purpose of the debut, but rather, in any case, its effect. It is a symbolic act. And it must not be confused with the practical murder of the parents, as it emerges in the fantasy of the rebellion. Furthermore, the act of appropriation of one's own life in the debut is a decisive act that can even drive a young person to fulfil their parents' desire. In such a case, their surrender is not a dependent or an adhesive act. The nucleus of that decisive act is the lived experience of responsibility, which breaks the adhesive infantile bond and instals an autonomous personal reference. And it coincides with the fall of the symbiotic infantile super-ego and with its replacement by an autonomous super-ego, along with the recombination of identifications and the emergence of personal desire.

The decision of the debut is simultaneous with a functional change of the super-ego. In that change, the syncretic prohibitions of the adhesion are replaced by generic rules that aim at the collective world, beyond the local symbiotic law. In that transformation, the ambiguity of the archaic super-ego – which is sustained in a syncretic bond and instals a possessive narcissism – is exchanged for a generic law that recognizes the desire of the self and of others.

Let us examine the following case. Agnes, a 13-year old girl, consulted about her activity of fantasizing. Her experience included two or three imaginary companions in her games and fantasies. The main one was called Avatar, an inseparable, good and unconditional companion. He was willing to do anything and would never let her down at difficult times. We can recognize in him the unconditional pre-Oedipal phallic figure, who provides for and completes the still narcissistic girl. He was quite the opposite to her feared figures – her female friends and her mother – whose demanding vigilance pursued her every time she let down her guard. These women could discover her fraud – who she really was – and that would end in a real catastrophe. She hid that, as she believed that she was surely abnormal and they were very intolerant. Here we note that the idealized imagoes and the persecutory super-ego are one and the same imago, seen from two different perspectives. Agnes pretended to be someone approved by the super-ego, as if it discovered the fraud, it would declare her abnormal. Moses and Eglé Laufer noted this fact in clinical work of the feeling of *abnormality* that could lead to suicide in extreme cases. The manic object, which sustained the latent self-esteem, becomes a cruel and persecutory object if the ideal is broken. Edith Jacobson defined that cruel object as the archaic super-ego. The juvenile rebellion establishes in a scene of real objects a symbolic event and "realizes" in them a murder that replaces the symbolic act of castration of the idealized pre-Oedipal object. In usual clinical practice, that event is expressed in the young person's disappointment with their parents, who "do not know or cannot," as Donald Meltzer notes. The infantile figures lose their ideal, sacred place and are transformed into ordinary human figures.

After some work, Agnes realized that those women thought the same as her. She believed that, in reality, she could not take an exam without failing it. And because of that she withdrew into her imaginary world. The fantasy was the refuge from a no way situation generated by her archaic super-ego. It is easy to note that her cruelty covered up her underlying idealization. Agnes had to undertake an intense work of de-idealization if she wanted to get out of that syncretic refuge, which had turned into a real prison.

School exams, the gaze of her female friends and her own mother replaced the surveillance of her archaic super-ego. She was just another avatar in a world of giants and imaginary figures who hid their true self. In turn, the fantasized world provided a focused, constant attention and a prosthetic solution for her need to be looked after. Here we note the confluence of the illusory protection of idealized figures and the concomitant possessive tyranny of a world that imprisons her.

Only a neutral analysis could reveal the reason for that unconditional need. Agnes presents the dilemma whenever her puberty brings into question the latent idealization and re-edits the problem between the desiring girl and the supposed possessor of that lack in being and possessing. She seeks to dominate access to an idealized wedding – primary scene – which supposedly enjoys those goods that are frustrated for the excluded daughter, or son, as the case may be. Fantasies of exclusion and of unjust frustration are the illusory defence against a fault that appears in the structure of the neurotic and that this person needs to overcome and accept if they are to be reconciled with their human condition.

***

The debut is not an isolated event in the life of an adolescent. It has a prehistory of a chain of events that usually occur around puberty. I will describe them using Bion's model on the containing–contained relationship. After the extreme emotional dependence of early childhood, sexual latency facilitates the development of the functions of the ego, based on its belonging to latent infantile institutions. This belonging provides a solid support and promotes adhesive identifications with the naturalized symbols of the family and community culture. In the institutional frame all is obvious, habitual, conservative and natural. Everyday events establish a sacred or consecrated way of seeing and living. The family frame houses the child's need for security and their protective emotional dependence. It provides shelter, it distributes the functional assistance that their incipient ego still requires and exercises its function with the naturality of the infantile world view – *Weltanschauung der Kinder*.

Of course, that worldview includes an implicit set of rules, imposed by the usual tradition that is deployed in family life. Its rules, sacred and inarguable, neutralize everything that can move its conservative vision, which favours the usual over the new. The silence of the frame is more active than it seems, as it brings into play an intense disavowal of what contradicts its sacred beliefs and the bases of its certainty. The disavowal comes with the structural splitting – known in the description of latency – whose primary purpose denies the existence and the consequences of parental sexual coitus that can generate a new reality alien to the sacred order.

As a result of the splitting and sexual disavowal, the latent frame is ordered on an immobile, sacred scene, crystalized on infantile beliefs. Those beliefs tend to be shared by parents and children, as they form a solid group whose family rites celebrate together their characterological convictions. That cohesive whole imposes its group bible on any attempt at the new, as it experiences that event as an attack on its homeostasis.

However, the frame is essential for the appearance of a new event that triggers the *adolescent debut*. The debut is a profane act that reinstates the use of sexuality, excluded by the latent sacred order, when the children were preserved from adult sexual desire. The latent Oedipal law split the nuptial sexual scene from infantile life. With it, sacralization increases. On that prehistory, the effective event of the debut must have enough emotional force to move the solid infantile world vision. If it does not achieve this, it will be absorbed and neutralized by its denial, which will reduce it to an unsubstantial, superficial or foolish event. The force of their emotion must generate a similar conviction to that described in Freud's experience regarding hysteria. Something makes a sign of a truth. And it shows the existence of a universe of meanings beyond their latent vision. Their discovery, after the event that made the sign – a truth that the young person discovers about their sex or about the life they experience – is embodied in their own who, and allows them to take control of their life and their future. From then on, they will have another angle of vision, distinct from that of their parents or that of their community. And from then on, they will see life with their own eyes.

That event marks an evolutionary crisis, with multiple changes in the content and in the functions of their psychic life. Particularly, in their identifications and in the function and quality of their super-ego. Their journey depends on the legitimization of the impulse of the desire and the strength of the super-ego. As, at the beginning – this is seen frequently with adolescents in clinical practice – the conflict between incipient desire and the latent frame runs the risk of going towards the tracks of the feeling of abnormality, when the latent super-ego qualifies as illegitimate or abnormal any desire different from their ideal. Improper desire threatens the young person, who thinks of themself as improper, a degenerate, abnormal, as Laufer described at the Brent Centre for Young People. It is no surprise that those cases end in serious guilt or persecutory crises, when the latent super-ego persecutes the user of the inappropriate desire and points it out as undesirable. The suicide impulse is not a depressive symptom or an object loss, as some believe they had discovered. It is a narcissistic collapse at the guilty presence of an anomalous – sexual – version of the ego, different from the ideal ego.

The other more frequent track legitimizes desire and gives the young person the right to question an established order. In that case, the legitimization makes a sign of a future decision and generates a change. The installation of the new desire needs something more than its intensity. It is necessary for a psychic agency to legitimize its existence. In general, such agency emerges in the *inter-est* of the family out of respect for the individuality of the blossoming person. Such *inter-est* – coined by Hannah Arendt – is perhaps the most human gesture that culture has achieved, in the form of a respect interested in the desire of the fellow person. Without that legitimization, the young person succumbs to the narcissistic myopia of those who cannot see further than their own emotional nose. And perhaps therein lies the fulcrum of the necessary lever to make those gestures – of respect for desire and personal decision based on this. If the *inter-est* does not appear in the family, society tends to help: in the understanding of a friend, of the peer group or of an institute assisting the family. Without them, the young adolescent is cast away to face their desire still outside of themselves and sees in it the risk of abnormality. The weight of the latent super-ego prejudices the voice of the juvenile desire and marginalizes it. From there it can only come out with the help of an *inter-est* that legitimizes it.

From this observation we can gather that the individual voice is never alone. It participates in a dialogue with the references that legitimize it, sustain it, criticize it and question it. The delicate balance of references sets the temperature and the distance that each young person has with their close ones and with those whom they know and wish to know on their horizon of expansion. The examination of the discourse shows a dialogue on two different planes: on the one hand, between the young person and those who accompany them in their discourse, and on the other hand, among the arguments and ideologies running through them – in their family, their community, their culture and their desires – and the language they use to translate and publish them.

Here we are not concerned with the specific content of those ideologies but rather the discursive position that they occupy in the process. The latent identifications group together around the institutions that infancy proposed. These instal themselves around the latent super-ego that offers a refuge for identifications and delegated functions. The function of the depository, coined by Pichon Rivière, allows us to understand the complete set of functions that that character performs throughout childhood and adolescence – of containment, regulation, opposition, guidance, refuge and deposit of the young person's undesired projections. At the heart of that relationship of depositing, a very solid tie of sustenance is maintained of the constants of usual life, which contribute to sustaining the most elemental narcissistic security of the young person and their family. That unconditional and narcissistic sustenance is the foundation on which the most convulsed processes of the debut unfold. That foundation has the value of a fixed, silent frame, in which the primary and intolerable anxieties of young people and their family are deposited, especially relationships with fantasies of betrayal, abandonment, orphanhood and the empty nest. These fantasies correspond to the infantile vision of the experience of separation and of differentiation that begin in the debut and end in the definitive individuation and subjectivation of each young person.

The sudden change in the mute frame of infancy into the whirlwind of the debut releases an enormous energy that was in potency in the adhesive infantile world. The primitive adhesions are exchanged for explosives and overblown gestures of liberation and rebellion. That superficial explosive climate is defensive. Its nature is similar to what occurred in the frame, as it maintains in silence a potential and highly feared break, in jeopardizing the prior status quo sustained by the ritual institution of the frame. And at the same time it is longed for, as it contains the underlying movement of subversion and of break that will culminate in the fall of the latent super-ego.

The dramatic double play of tensions illustrates the polyphonic character of the adolescent process – in being immersed in the communities of the family world and the peer group – and especially the dialectic character of that coupling between the tensions of the debut and the resistances of the latent frame, which finally lead to overcoming – *Aufhebung* – those and the synthesis of the conflict. The young person is dis-alienated from that which they fragmented and projected on their close ones and on the material objects that surrounded them and which they consumed. And they accept their human condition, in accepting the conflicts and contradictions of their life and of their dramatic relationship with their surroundings.

The defences against the pain associated with this *Aufhebung* shift the human drama to the world of things and alter the emotion typical of desire towards objectified appetites, in which the thirst for dominance prevails over sexual desire. The thirst for dominance is directed especially at one's own desire – as this is still seen as an alien and uncontrollable danger – and pacifies them as they transform it into a success-based skill, where the emotion becomes a mere pleasure of conquest. The case of Agnes provides a good example of this defence. The objectification of her fellows – transformed into objects of conquest and consumption – reverts onto her ego and alters her emotionality. Many times, that path has no return from the objectified world, due to the transformation of the emotions into mere bodily and narcissistic sensations. An adhesive and potentially addictive condition is added to the relationship with her fellow people, displaced to a relationship with objectified objects or people. The rich human drama becomes a bundle of simple, proto-colar and characterological relationships, with dominated or fetishized objects.

The emotion's drift to objectified relationships makes the human being lose their rich polyphony. It is degraded into an impoverished dialogue where only dominance matters – of themself and the other – in a mono-tonous, protocolized relationship, close to the ritual, due to the intense control of a feared freedom. That degradation concludes in a syncretic conduct, without symbolic flair, in which imaginative and intelligible possibilities are contracted to the miniscule superficiality of a mindless belonging to a group or institution. In that case, the groupality – which is essential as a juvenile scenario – loses its adolescent condition and becomes an antisocial gang. Their antisocial attitude is not necessarily a rebellion against the law, but a challenge to humanity, whose emotional fragility is lived as a weakness from their arrogance of their supposed superficial superiority.

Note

1 *Aufhebung*: G.W.F. Hegel (1807), in *Die Phänomenologie des Geistes* (*Phenomenology of Spirits*) used this term to indicate the better argument that annuls and conserves the opposites of the dialectic antithesis. The German verb *aufheben* has the double meaning of conserving and eliminating something and the noun *Aufhebung* retains that ambiguity.

References

Avenburg, R. (1973). *La identidad en el adolescente*. Buenos Aires: Paidós/Asociación Argentina de Psiquiatría y Psicología de la Infancia y la Adolescencia.

Bleger, J. (1971). *La identidad del adolescente. Fundamentos y tipicidad*. Official report to the Second Argentine Congress on Child and Youth Psychopathology, 21–24 October 1971, Buenos Aires, Argentina. Buenos Aires: Paidós/Asociación Argentina de Psiquiatría y Psicología de la Infancia y la Adolescencia.

Blos, P. (1962). *On Adolescence: A Psychoanalytic Interpretation*. New York: Free Press.

Cahn, R. (1991). Du sujet. *Revue française psychanalyse* 55: 1371–1490.

Cahn, R. et al. (2016). *Le sujet dans la psychanalyse aujourd'hui*. Paris: Presses Universitaires de France.

Gutton, P. (1996). L'école française de psychanalyse de l'adolescent. In: Marty, F. (ed.) *L'Adolescence*. Paris: Collège International de L'Adolescence.

Hegel, G.H.F. (1807). *Die Phänomenologie des Geistes*.

Jacobson, E. (1954). *The Self and the Object World*. New York: International Universities Press.

Moguillansky, C. (2012). Las instituciones latentes y el debut adolescente. *Controversias en Psicoanálisis de niños y adolescentes* 10. Available at www.controversiasonline.apdeba.org.

7 Braving the erotic field in the treatment of adolescents

Mary Brady

I find my patient's body – and my body – to be more directly the subjects of analysis with adolescents than with adults or with younger children. Erotic transference and countertransference can be particularly fraught because of the intensity of emergent bodily sensations in the adolescent and because of her or his normal developmental immaturity. Adolescents need help to name and integrate their newfound bodily experiences. Their minds need to grow into the bodies they now inhabit. It is a challenge for analysts to talk about feelings the adolescent has barely begun to name. Indeed, budding sexuality and the memories and feelings it stirs in us of our own sexual beginnings are no small things to metabolise. And yet, with rare exceptions, the area of erotic transference/countertransference in the treatment of adolescents is largely ignored in analytic writing.[1]

The catastrophic prospect of boundary violations, particularly with minors, can lead to a timid avoidance of the erotic in our work with adolescents, yielding what I term an 'erotic insufficiency.' The analyst can fear exploiting the trust necessary for an adolescent to bring his or her emerging sexuality into analysis in a lively manner. Feelings that arouse the greatest conflict and guilt in the analyst are precisely those that are most vulnerable to our defensive rejection. In order to consider these ideas I will relate a period in the analysis of a 12-year-old boy when the erotic transference and countertransference were at a height. I will also suggest that the terms erotic transference and erotic countertransference do not fully capture the intensely interactional nature of these experiences. I suggest 'erotic field' better conveys this fluidity.

Erotic transference and countertransference with younger children can seem comparatively comfortable.[2] An eight-year-old boy fantasised that he was a king, and I, his golden-haired queen, living in a castle together, and that we would never have to part. While the scene I am describing is only the most conscious aspect of a deeper fantasy, I believe that there are also other reasons why my countertransference response was comparatively easy to bear. I could feel the poignancy of this idyllic picture, and sympathise with my patient's frustrations at the inescapable realities of life, such as how old one is, and how old are one's analyst, mother, father, and so on – and how

DOI: 10.4324/9781003380283-7

much these exigencies determine. In this familiar oedipal scene, one cannot have what one wants and yet it is better to have wanted it. However, it was also my young patient's age and related physical immaturity that contributed to a less charged erotic transference – countertransference than with adolescent patients.

Changing bodies, changing minds

The body of the adolescent is changing radically before his or her own eyes, as well as before mine. Adolescent boys can shoot up a foot in height over a couple of years. Brian, aged 13, encountered me in the hallway before a session and said, "Have you always been that short?" His body was new in many ways, and led to new experiences in relation to himself, me and everyone else. Brian and I experienced together his pubertal development and the meanings it shifted within our relationship.

Naomi, a pubertal girl, having had the puberty/sex talk at school that day, asked me with utter sincerity: "What's puberty for?" I was struck that though I could answer the question in a limited biological sense, the larger psychological and emotional meanings would take years to comprehend.

Evelyn, a 16-year-old in analysis spoke about being on the verge of having intercourse with her boyfriend. I asked her, "Do you think having sex will change anything inside you or between us?" At first she demurred, but soon said that, "Having intercourse will be the end of childhood." Something would definitively change inside her, as well as between us, and between her and her parents. She would cross a line from her child bodily self to an adult bodily self and there would no longer be a substantive divide between her experiences and those of adults in a sexual sense. Experience would be gained, but a precious boundary that allowed some element of childhood to remain (all too scarce for this girl) would be lost.

Around this time Evelyn asked to use the couch. Her 'use' of the couch[3] was different than any I have experienced. She was in constant motion and reminded me of a seal. She would flip from side to side and then flip over on her stomach to look at me. My experience was of not being able to think with all this motion and I wished Evelyn would just lie still. Evelyn was giving me an experience of how much commotion she felt inside and how unsettled she felt in her body during this stage of her development.

Evelyn asked to use the couch in order to talk about sexuality. My agreement for her to lie down evoked intimate and erotic feelings in her towards me. Soon after starting to use the couch she told me of making out with her boyfriend in his car for the first time. She said: "I found myself tracing your initials in the steam on the window." As we explored this action it seemed that I was both present in Evelyn's erotic feelings *and* that she was summoning me to help her create some 'brakes' to allow thinking space while making out with her boyfriend.

In all of these instances, the teens experienced rapid bodily changes that they brought to analysis for consideration. I will turn briefly to erotic transference and countertransference in the psychoanalytic literature on adults in order to create a backdrop from which to consider the far more scant literature on transference–countertransference with adolescents.

Erotic transference and countertransference in the adult literature

Person defines "erotic transference" as interchangeable with "transference love", meaning "some mixture of tender, erotic, and sexual feelings that a patient experiences in reference to his or her analyst and, as such, forms part of a positive transference" (Person, 1985: 161).[4] She describes the erotic transference as "both goldmine and minefield" (1985: 163). Passionate feelings are likely to be confusing to patient and analyst and thus their consideration can yield great rewards. Simultaneously, intense feelings in the patient or analyst are also prone to either acting out or defensive avoidance.

A patient's erotic feelings toward an analyst can be intensely driven and even psychotic in the Kleinian sense of losing touch with reality. Blum (from a different theoretical viewpoint) describes 'eroticized transference' as a "... particular species of erotic transference, an extreme sector of a spectrum. It is an intense, vivid, irrational, erotic preoccupation with the analyst, characterized by overt, seemingly ego-syntonic demands for love and sexual fulfillment from the analyst" (Blum, 1973: 63).

In my experience there are patients who also waver between a *capacity* to experience strong feelings toward their analyst but who may lose hold of reality considerations in the throes of intense feelings.

Person points out that (even in the adult literature) erotic transference "has always been tainted by unsavory associations and continues to be thought of as slightly disreputable" (Person, 1985: 163) compared with analytic reflection on other forms of transference. In one sense this is strange, as Freud struggled mightily (in introducing his concept of infantile sexuality) to help us to see that intense and passionate forces are in us all from the beginning. And yet, perhaps we have to accept that passionate and deeply rooted forces always create some defensive alarm. How much more so when the patient has not reached adulthood?

In a well-known and ground-breaking paper, Searles (1959) squared off against the orthodox notion, prevalent at the time, that intense emotional reactions on the part of the analyst are pathological. He proposed three hypotheses:

> ... a) in the course of a successful psychoanalysis, the analyst goes through a phase of reacting to, and eventually relinquishing, the patient as being his oedipal love-object; b) in normal personality-development, the parent reciprocates the child's oedipal love with greater intensity than we have recognized heretofore; and c) in such normal development,

the passing of the Oedipus complex is at least as important a phase in ego-development as in superego development.

(Searles, 1959: 180)

Racker (1953) likewise contended that the Oedipus complex will express itself in every countertransference, while the form, consciousness of it and intensity vary:

... sometimes the analyst loves the patient genitally and desires her genital love towards him; he hates her if she then loves another man, feels rivalry of this man and jealousy and envy (heterosexual and homosexual) of their sexual pleasure. Sometimes he hates her if she hates him, and loves her if she suffers, for in this case he is revenged for the oedipic deceit. He feels satisfaction when the transference is very positive, but also castration anxiety and guilt feelings toward the husband, etc.

(Racker, 1953: 316)

I am using countertransference here to denote the analyst's experience of an intensely interactional transference–countertransference dialogue (Greenberg & Mitchell, 1983; Langs, 1981; Little, 1951; Ogden, 1997; Racker, 1957; 1958; Winnicott, 1949).[5]

Erotic transference and countertransference, adolescent style

Lena, discussing the erotic transference of a 16-year-old boy to his female therapist, contends:

Given the centrality of sexual impulses and fantasies in adolescence, one would think that the erotic transference is a common phenomenon in many therapists with adolescents ... When discussing this topic with colleagues working with adolescents most psychotherapists could think of cases when powerful sexual feelings coloured the transference relationship. And yet little has been written about the erotic transference in childhood and adolescence, even less about the experience of the therapist.

(Lena, 2017: 43)

Atkinson and Gabbard likewise comment: "erotic material in an adolescent's transference may create in the analyst a level of concern or even fear of parental retaliation should the parents become aware of the material" (1995: 174). I would add that the fear of parents' potential response can also be a projection of the analyst's own parental superego, which can lead to repression or avoidance.

Alvarez's (2012) work, "Types of sexual transference and countertransference in work with children and adolescents", is a rare and substantive contribution to this topic. She distinguishes amongst 'perverse' 'disordered' and 'normal' sexual transferences in children and adolescents. 'Perverse' denotes a dangerously addictive sexuality with sadistic and masochistic elements. 'Disordered' indicates an addictive but not fully perverse sexuality. And by 'normal' Alvarez denotes the child or adolescent's desire "to make someone's eyes light up" (Alvarez, 2012, p. 126) and "the need for a responsive interested object capable of being delighted" (ibid., p. 126).

Paton discusses a scenario in which an adolescent sexualises the therapeutic atmosphere to "avoid feelings of unhappiness and vulnerability" (Paton, 2017: 28) which would be similar to Blum's description of eroticised transference and could overlap with Alvarez's perverse or disordered sexual transferences.

Jackson (a male analyst) describes an 18-year-old woman's reaction to using the couch:

> For the first few weeks Sarah seemed tense, lying on the couch with her knees up as if she felt like a terrified virgin on her wedding night. This was poignantly represented when she told me how her new travel card gave her freedom to go wherever she wanted but left her worrying about whether she could manage the increased cost. She was able to recognise how the 'cost' in the transference connected in part to the increased access she had to her fantasies about my 'private life' and her hatred of feeling so excluded from it.
>
> (Jackson, 2017: 18)

Jackson (2017) warns that when sexuality emerges within the transference and countertransference with our adolescent patients: "... threatening to disrupt our thinking and shatter our psychic equilibrium ... we should not underestimate our propensity to avoid, negate and defend ourselves against these dynamics, even when we are conscious of them" (ibid.: 6).

He notes that it can be difficult to distinguish between being safe and containing of our adolescent patients' erotic feelings and "something that is rationalised as safe and containing but which is essentially evasive and defensive on the part of the therapist" (ibid.: 12). Similarly, Atkinson and Gabbard (1995) describe an erotic transference of a male patient with a female therapist and note that the therapist in such a pairing may be tempted to overemphasise maternal feelings.

Just as we may be avoidant of erotic feelings in clinical work with adolescents, we also seem to be avoidant of these feelings in clinical writing. Jackson notes that while the analytic literature on erotic transference countertransference with adults is thin, "it is especially thin in relation to psychoanalytic work with children and adolescents" (Jackson, 2017: 8).

Adolescent treatment requires a freedom to experience and tolerate intense feelings, while attempting to neither over-stimulate nor neglect sexual feelings. The following vignette is an excellent example of this: Jackson describes his response when Sarah, who he sometimes feels to be the "apple of my eye" (Jackson, 2017, p. 18) tells him that she has kissed a close friend of her boyfriend:

> The intensity of the impact this had on me was startling. I experienced it like a personal assault – a body blow, affecting my whole physiology and evoking something not far off a sense of outrage as if she had actually been unfaithful to me.
>
> (ibid.: 18)

The intensity of Jackson's reaction jarred him and gradually led him to understand that Sarah had experienced their recent agreement for her to use the couch as a sexual enactment. Jackson's subsequent vacation break had thus felt like a betrayal to her. As he reflected on his intense reaction Jackson became more active in interpreting how his breaks, "could feel like a violation of the therapy and the therapeutic relationship" (ibid.: 18). Sarah then tells him that she had kissed the boy to hurt him more than her boyfriend. Jackson replies:

> I acknowledged the importance of what she was saying about how angry, jealous and cheated on she felt by me over Easter, adding that perhaps now I needed to know what that was like – including what it was like to feel sexually jealous.
>
> (ibid.: 18)

Jackson keeps a close eye to the effect of his comments on his patient. While always important, this close attunement to how our words are experienced is only more important in this erotic territory – over-stimulating or insufficient?

Erotic insufficiency/erotic playback

The emerging bodily experiences of the adolescent (first menstruation, first wet dream, first masturbation to orgasm, and so on) are parts of a "virgin territory" (Holtzman & Kulish, 1997; Kulish, 1998). For the analyst, the patient's pubertal development can rouse feelings of venturing into a particularly taboo, forbidden, loaded, and vulnerable area. This can create hesitancy and inhibition in the analyst, making her less likely to be able to stand for the acceptance and containment of these sensations and emotions.

Samuels (a post-Jungian analyst) suggests that:

> … the subtle damage and deprivation caused by erotic deficit is far less spoken of than what is caused by erotic excess. Physical incest takes place at an appallingly high frequency … but something equally central and much more benevolent in sexuality is being overlooked.
>
> (Samuels, 2000: 278)

I prefer the term 'erotic insufficiency' as deficit implies a lack of capacity, while therapists' avoidance of the erotic is often caused more by discomfort and anxiety than incapacity.

Samuels describes 'erotic playback' in parenting and in clinical processes:

> In the family this is the way in which the parent communicates to children of both sexes that they are admirable, physically desirable and erotically viable creatures. Of course, in a family or in analysis I am referring only to incest fantasy and not to the physical enactment of such fantasy.
>
> (ibid.: 277)

Samuels adds that the erotic includes more than sex, it also encompasses: "harmony, relatedness, purpose, significance, and meaning: Eros ... This means, of course, that ambivalence, anxiety, jealousy, rivalry, and a sense of lack will also be present" (ibid.: 278). To translate into my Bionian clinical language, an analyst would need to be able to be emotionally responsive and containing to the erotic (in a broad sense) in a patient and also to all of the related subtleties and problems – what's too much, what's too blank or defensive? What is hard to bear about the erotic? What is enlivening or even transformative?

Samuels concept of 'erotic playback' is not simplistic. He sees sexual identity as not "unified, fixed, static, eternal, universal" (ibid.: 278). Erotic playback encourages the individual "to think of himself or herself in a diversified way, to come alive and hold together in the mind all aspects of the self – body areas ..." (ibid.: 278) Samuels acknowledges that erotic playback is vulnerable to mis-attunement as well as more egregious failures.

Ogden's work on the 'aliveness' of the analytic exchange broadly approximates what Samuels is describing. Ogden describes the analyst's "spontaneity and freedom to respond to the analysand from his own experience in the analytic situation in a way that is not strangulated by stilted caricatures of analytic neutrality" (Ogden, 1995: 696). He says:

> ... every form of psychopathology represents a specific type of limitation of the individual's capacity to be fully alive as a human being. The goal of analysis from this point of view is larger than that of the resolution of unconscious intrapsychic conflict, the diminution of symptomatology, the enhancement of reflective subjectivity and self-understanding, and the increase of sense of personal agency. Though one's sense of being alive is intimately intertwined with each of the above-mentioned capacities, I believe that the experience of aliveness is a quality that is superordinate to these capacities.
>
> (Ogden, 1995: 696)

More specific to the present discussion, Elise defines 'analytic eroticism' as the "aesthetic capacity to keep ... embodied vitality alive in the analytic relationship" (Elise, 2017: 34). She compares analytic eroticism to Kristeva's (2014) discussion of maternal eroticism:

> The encounter with the mother as erotic being brings into being the child's erotic self, both in the specifically sexual and in the most general sense: vitality in living, a curious and creative engagement with life – Eros.
>
> (Elise, 2017: 34)

A simple and lovely example comes to mind. Seven-year-old Spencer came to his session dressed in a collared shirt instead of his usual tee-shirt. He told me it had been 'picture day' at school and that his mother told him he was wearing his 'handsome' shirt. How beautifully, naturally and subtly she was sowing the seeds of his developing sense of being an attractive and desirable boy and future man.

As parents or analysts we do not often consciously set out to provide our children or patients 'erotic playback'. Perhaps we have trouble naming that along with the growth of the mind, we also hope to help free the growth of erotic aliveness in our patients – both sexually and in related forms, such as a passion for ideas, rich sensuality, and a broad and complex range of emotional experience and expressiveness.

Timid avoidance of erotic feelings in the consulting room deprives adolescents of sincere adult thinking in relation to the challenges of enjoying and managing sexual feelings. The analyst's capacity to be aware of his or her erotic feelings but not to act on them comes across in many ways. If the analyst can feel some ease with sexual feelings alive in the field, then his or her own, as well as the patient's capacity to think about sensual/bodily/sexual feelings may develop. Of course, this sounds easy in the abstract, but is not so easy in the heat of the moment.

Clinical example – 'pick-up' sticks

Frank, a sensitive 12-year-old boy with a 'cool', teenage demeanour, appeared at least two years older than his actual age. He was in analysis for depression following his father's death. His mother was depressed and collapsed in relation to her husband's illness and death, but also suffered from a more chronic depression which had predated this event. Now two years into the analysis, Frank's depression had diminished and an erotic transference developed, partly under the pressure of puberty, and also in response to our having begun a fourth weekly session. Frank had agreed to a fourth session because he could see that our work was helping him to use his mind more actively to sort out his feelings from his mother's feelings. He had observed: "When my mother is depressed I feel like I can feel her feelings." His mother accepted my recommendation of a fourth session because she was concerned both about Frank's painful stutter and about some of Frank's 'risky' friends.[6]

Frank felt that I had a special interest in him as demonstrated by my wanting to see him so often. He at first complained that the fourth session was too much time and took away from other things. However, at one point I noted aloud that he seemed distant following my having been away. I commented: "It's easy to feel if someone is not there, that they don't care about you." He replied: "I know you care about me because of the fourth session." This was the end of the hour, and before he got up he touched my leg with one of the pick-up sticks we had been playing with and commented that my stockings were "shiny." I am reminded of Freud's (1915: 169) comment in "Observations on Transference Love" that the analyst "has evoked this love by instituting analytic treatment in order to cure the neurosis".

At times I noticed Frank looking at my breasts.[7] Another time he looked at my legs and asked, "Are they stockings?" I said, "Guys your age are often curious about girls' things, like stockings and underwear. Another thing about your age is that there are a lot of intense changes in one's body that can often feel hard to talk about." Frank replied with emotion, "I know what you mean. I'm beginning to have acne and other people my age aren't getting it yet."

In another session Frank touched my wedding ring and asked:

F: What stone is it?
A: You may be wondering not just what stone, but what the ring means.
F: That you're married.
A: Maybe, but then there's also what that means to you because you're pretty close to me.
F: Have you seen the movie *When Harry Met Sally*? The man in the movie didn't notice the woman at first.
A: You are noticing girls more in general but also noticing me in that way.

It was near the end of the session and Frank was tracing the veins in his forearm with his finger. I was struck by the change in his forearm over the two years I had seen him – his forearm had changed from that of a boy to that of a man. At this moment I felt attracted to him in the same way as I might toward an adult, masculine man. At 12 he had already largely developed the body of a man. It has often been observed that it is a challenge for girls who menstruate early to integrate their experiences, having had less time for antecedent emotional and cognitive development. It is also true for boys who have the bodies of men without the same psychological development.

Frank hummed the wedding march under his breath another day, and more than once slipped and asked why we had not met on the fifth day, on which we did not have an appointment. I pointed out he might be wishing we met that day as well. I mentioned the possibility of a fifth session to his mother, who spoke of it to her brother. Frank's mother and uncle seemed to have an underlying suspicion regarding my interest in Frank. Indeed, I had to struggle to sort out my own feelings of attraction to Frank to keep myself from withdrawing from him due to anxiety about my erotic countertransference.

The following interchange seems to capture the incestuous aspects of the transference, and the anxieties surrounding it:

F: I was reading about a bank robber who got shot nine times, shot through the mouth, tongue, teeth. With leprosy could you have a finger fall off?

A: Where did you hear about that possibility?

F: In history class. I think it could happen.

A: It reminds me of an old wives' tale that if a guy masturbates enough his penis could fall off. It's not true, but I guess it comes from that part of a guy's body being really important to him (Frank nods) and worrying something could happen to it.

F: In drama class today we were done with work, so we were just chilling, and somebody raised the story of a teacher, who had sex with her 12-year-old student, and he got her pregnant. She was married and had three children. She went to jail, and when she got out, he got her pregnant again.

A: What did you think about that story?

F: It's weird, 24 years older is a little bit of a problem – she was 36. (Frank trails off).

A: Maybe you're uncomfortable talking about it, as I'm an older woman you're close to, and you're 12.

Frank was unable to say any more about this issue, but I felt that it crystallised the transference–countertransference situation. I told him, "I don't think it was good what happened between the teacher and student, but I wouldn't want you to think such feelings are weird." I gulped internally as I linked this loaded story about the teacher and the boy directly to our relationship. There had been many indicators of Frank's feelings, so it did not feel premature. I also felt that I was not being seductive, but naming something implicit to make it more explicit.

Sometimes there could be reasons to allow material to continue to evolve in derivative form, whereas at other times it could feel over-stimulating to make a direct link to the analytic couple. As I look back many years later, this comment has a feeling of rightness to me. The situation in the room *was* stimulating – a boy going through puberty and an older woman. I felt attracted to Frank as I might to a man – and experienced an ordinary preoccupation with these feelings and a wishfulness. My private internal sexual fantasy included the sense of an older, more sexually experienced woman with a virile, but unexperienced young boy/man. Of course, I was also well aware that Frank was not actually a young man, but a boy. I believe that my ways of relating to Frank in the hours of his analytic sessions always kept this in mind, but that the transitions occurring within in him were stimulating to both of us.

Soon after, Frank told me that his uncle asked: "Did your analyst propose yet?" Frank said, "It's weird you want me to come so much, since most people go once or twice a week." I said: "Sometimes people are uncomfortable with positive feelings, but I imagine you felt confused about whose ideas to be loyal to." Frank nodded. He seemed to register that sharing and understanding his loving and sexual feelings could be helpful to him. I think that my effort to tolerate erotic feelings toward Frank, despite these accusations and my own discomfort, helped Frank to tolerate and integrate his own sexual and romantic feelings more fully.

Discussion

My comments to Frank were intended to have an open-ended "unsaturated" (Bion, 1962) quality, in order to allow Frank's feelings, thoughts and experiences to develop further. An analyst has to be willing to brave this territory if she expects her patient to likewise be able to. While it is often useful to proceed in an unsaturated manner, it is especially true in relation to the physical changes of adolescence. The bodily changes and sensations of adolescence are so big that they can only be taken in gradually.

When helping an adolescent to name erotic feelings, we are also indirectly implying certain attitudes towards sexuality – that it's there, that sexuality is part of us, that even very intense feelings can be shared. When I look back at this material it seems right to me that I did not interpret Frank's story about the teacher in relation to incestuous feelings towards his mother, (while of course there would be an element of truth to this). Such a genetic interpretation would have been avoidant of the erotic feelings in the room and could have signalled to Frank my unwillingness to be close to his feelings.

An analyst might not directly interpret derivative material in some situations. The "perverse" children described by Alvarez (2012, p. 122) might take such an interpretation in an addictive direction and be unable to use it to think. Sexually over-stimulated or abused adolescents might be better served by discussing sexuality in more derivative form, as they have too often been victim to sexuality crashing through. Over-concrete children, such as those on the Autism Spectrum, would be unlikely to use an explicit transference interpretation fluidly, rendering such comments useless or confusing. Also, a therapist must consider the level of preparatory groundwork that might allow intense feelings to be addressed more directly. Frank had already been in analysis for two years when erotic feelings emerged and we had weathered some other storms.

Of course analysts must always observe reactions to what we have said and have an attitude of humility that while we may have intended a comment one way, it may be experienced in another. It is my impression that interpreting this material to Frank more explicitly was useful. Leaving these feelings unnamed could imply that they were too catastrophic to identify. Instead, very loaded feelings were named and the boundaries and purposes of our work remained in place.

Retrospectively, the erotic transference–countertransference with Frank emerged at a specific time in the treatment and has been more in the background subsequently. Shortly after my patient's erotic transference reached a height (at age 13), he started a romantic relationship with a girl his age. She remained his girlfriend for the next two years. Across this time I was impressed with Frank's growing ability to talk directly with her about his feelings.

I believe that the erotic transference experienced with an emotionally available but safe object became a launching ground for Frank's own erotic life. I thought that his experience of having a single object who was paying attention to him, and to whom he was paying attention, allowed for a deepening of an impressive capacity for intimate feelings. Frank's mother's depression likely made "the potentiating capacity of eroticism" (Elise, 2017: 35) more important in the analytic relationship than it might have been had these feelings been more reciprocally available in a parental relationship.

Adolescents frequently present with bravado, which masks their developmental unreadiness for some experiences. I believe that the period of erotic transference–countertransference allowed Frank a trying-on of feelings and fantasies, as well as some room to verbalise these experiences. Adolescent treatment often has this quality – a dress rehearsal[8] is allowed for issues that feel unsafe – either for reasons of conflict, or developmental unreadiness. Adolescents often experience first love with an unavailable object, but growth is happening meanwhile.

My experience of Frank's erotic transference is much as Searles described it in "Oedipal love in the countertransference" (Searles, 1959). That is, that the child accepts that his oedipal strivings are unrealisable not primarily through fear of and identification with the forbidding rival parent, but instead:

> ... through the ego strengthening experience of finding that the beloved parent reciprocates his love – responds to him, that is, as being a worthwhile and lovable, individual, as being, indeed, a conceivably desirable love partner – and renounces him only with an accompanying sense of loss on the parent's own part ... This child emerges ... with his ego strengthened out of the knowledge that his love, however unrealizable, is reciprocated.
>
> (Searles, 1959: 188)

Concomitantly, emotional dulling can occur if the "beloved parent had to repress his or her reciprocal desire for the child, chiefly through the mechanism of unconscious denial of the child's importance to the parent" (ibid.: 189).

Davies, an American Relational analyst suggests that erotic transference can be infantilized and seen only in pre-oedipal or oedipal dimensions. She suggests that as infantile conflicts are understood, then "the rich efflorescence, not the disappearance of passionate desire in the analytic relationship" often ensues (Davies, 1998: 752). Within the "relatively safe confines of the analytic space ... there is a freedom to experience those aspects of sexual desire and erotic fantasy that are part of emergent self-experiences" (ibid.: 752).

Davies relates a riveting moment from her own family life, which she felt informed her understanding of emergent adolescent sexuality. Davies and her husband were engrossed in a conversation when their daughters (who had been playing dressing up) ran by. The 12-year-old:

> ... had piled her long dark hair on top of her head and had put on a clingy black jersey, slit up the side. The outfit was completed with black fishnet stockings, patent-leather high heels and a red garter. I was astounded, but her father let slip an almost imperceptible but still subliminally audible gasp – a gasp heard loud and clear by his very vulnerable daughter woman and her then immobilized, but horrified, mother. In a series of microseconds, meaningful looks of danger and confusion ricocheted spitfire around this now palpable triangle, and my daughter, crying hysterically, ran from the room.
>
> (Davies, 1998: 759)

Gathering himself, Davies' husband went to talk to his daughter. Later, equilibrium apparently restored, Davies asked what he had said to accomplish this:

> "I told her the truth," he said, "that I had never seen her looking so beautiful before ... in such a grown-up way ... that it had taken my breath away ... that I liked it ... but that it was something I was going to have to get used to." "Did she say anything?" I asked. "No, but she smiled the most beautiful smile." And then he smiled.
>
> (Davies, 1998: 760)

Davies suggests that her husband's honest acknowledgement allows a 'beginning recognition' of adolescent emergent sexual subjectivity. The adolescent can experience being the object of another's sexual response in a reasonably titrated manner when that response feels both forthright and contained. I was struck by the pauses in her husband's speech, which Davies represented three times by '...'. These pauses seem to me a helpful communication in themselves, as they imply that one can pause and stop to think when in the midst of tumultuous feelings.

The analyst of an adolescent must be able to withstand a series of anxieties in relation to sexuality – for instance, "Is what we're talking about too much?", "Is it too exciting?", "Is my interest too voyeuristic?" – in order to help the adolescent tolerate her or his own excitements and anxieties. This willingness to tread in an anxiety-provoking area can hopefully lend what I call 'erotic sufficiency' to our work with adolescents. Davies suggests:

... analysts' ability to contain their own desire with self-awareness equates to parents' observance of the incest prohibition. Such self-conscious containment creates and protects a gap in which the patient's subjectivity can come into its own.

(Davies, 1998: 59)

Lombardi (2017) comments:

Adolescence involves confrontation with a *choice* that becomes decisive for all subsequent development: this choice consists of either facing up to adolescent turbulence or mobilizing all possible strategies to avoid it.

(Lombardi, 2017: 113)

This period of treatment felt turbulent to me as well as, I imagine, to Frank. While I do not feel I was inappropriate or flirtatious in the sessions, outside of the hours we spent together in his psychotherapy I thought I must be losing my mind to have strong feelings of attraction to a 12/13-year-old. In retrospect, I think that Frank and I were able to sustain turbulence without closing it down too quickly, yielding an 'erotic sufficiency.'

Erotic field

My work with Frank took place a decade and a half ago when I was still a candidate in child analysis. As I reflect on it now, I am struck that my experience with Frank was of a "bi-personal field" (Baranger & Baranger, 2008; Molinari, 2017), "analytic third" (Ogden, 1994) or "intermediate area of experience" (Winnicott, 1971) though my Freudian supervision did not employ these terms. My experience was of a continuous exchange of emotional elements that through dreams and narratives (such as the 12-year-old impregnating his 36 year-old teacher) "find a way of expressing and narrating what is going on in the depths of the relational exchange" (Ferro, 1999: 158).

Shared meanings and feelings could be elaborated with Frank in a way that did not have to be too pinned down. Meanings could continually take shape from a shared (though not, on my part, an explicitly expressed) experience of erotic and romantic longings. These longings could also come into contact with a reality of limits in the relationship and the allowance that these longings be transformed for other purposes, such as Frank's assumption of his romantic and erotic life. It is interesting that while coming from a Freudian view that emphasised the intra-psychic, my supervisor seemed entirely comfortable with this way of working.

The supervision[9] I was engaged in during his psychotherapy with me was instrumental in helping me not to inhibit erotic feelings in my relationship with Frank. The use of a consultant may be particularly important at such times to help to think while feeling and to feel while thinking. In the context of the above clinical moment I recall my supervisor saying that it was good that I liked males, implying that Frank did not have to be deprived of the subtle ways this would come across in my interactions with him. I am reminded of Elise's comment:

> … what of the analyst's libidinal investment in that unique patient, in that analysis. An analysis cannot rest on the patient's libidinal energies alone. We might think of erotic energy as circulating in multiple directions in the intersubjective field of an analysis – a libidinally alive matrix…. A clinical situation of vibrancy can foster patients' increased libidinal investment in *themselves.*
>
> (Elise, 2017: 49).[10]

It is interesting to consider how the work with Frank might have been different with a heterosexual male analyst or a gay or lesbian analyst. It is important for all analysts to be able to be fluid and imaginative in experiencing ourselves as male or female, father or mother, or potentially in a homosexual or heterosexual role with a patient. Still, it seems to me at times that the specific genders of the pair are important, and perhaps especially so at puberty. Some early adolescent female patients relate to me as if I may be able to help them figure out the mysteries that are befalling them – after all I have gone through the bodily changes they are going through. In the current clinical material, the constellation of a heterosexual boy in early adolescence and a heterosexual female analyst may have allowed a particularly intense version of feelings that surely would have also been present in some form with this patient and a different analyst.

The terms 'erotic transference' and 'erotic countertransference' seem to me too static to capture the fluidity, subtlety or complexity that is better conveyed in the dynamic concept of an 'erotic field.' Hartmann, in a memorial paper for Muriel Dimen, highlights her complex use of field theory. He says: "Better to speak to/in the erotic field than to codify it as the patient's 'erotic transference'. To reify the transference is to forget that 'recursively, to reflect on desire and to contain it, enhance each other' (Dimen, 2011, p. 59)" (in Hartmann, 2017: 133).

When I think back to the period in my work with Frank when erotic feelings were in the forefront, it feels almost impossible to say, 'whose feeling is it?' Frank experienced my recommendation of frequent sessions as a possible seduction. His looking at my body was stimulating to me. I think of the complexity of a single moment - such as the one when Frank traced the veins on his forearm, and I felt attracted to him in a similar way as I might to an adult, masculine man. These were my feelings, located in me and unspoken. Nevertheless at the same time, his subtle and un-self-conscious action might represent a new sensuality and budding awareness of his body that I was also reacting to.

At times feelings might belong mainly to one member of the analytic couple. Frank felt frustrated that I did not let him in on my private life. But even such an experience, that was mainly his, includes a whole history of familial boundary experiences for both patient and analyst. Such personal experience of boundaries would necessarily in some way become part of the erotic field.

Conclusion

Analytic work with adolescents brings words like 'visceral', 'intense', 'in motion' and 'palpable' to mind. At times adolescents have been considered poorly suited for analytic treatment (Freud, 1958).[11] The changing body of the adolescent patient presents particular challenges to containment and pressures toward enactment in the treatment of adolescents. Lombardi, commenting on Ferrari (2004), notes: "a lack of experience with the adult world establishes the necessity for the adolescent to 'act in order to know'" (Lombardi, 2016: 4). When analysis can help an adolescent to understand and contain their bodily and familial changes, the bodily-based psycho-pathologies (eating disorders, cutting, substance abuse), which are characteristic disturbances of adolescence (Anderson, 2004; Brady, 2016) may be prevented or mitigated.

As I complete this paper, I think about its title. Is it 'entering' the erotic field with the adolescent patient or some other verb: what about 'surviving' or 'tolerating' or 'enjoying' or 'playing in' or 'braving?' As I mull over these verbs, they all have some element of truth, but 'braving' seems the most fitting – and thus the title changes … I will end this paper with Alvarez's reminder that: "Sometimes the positive transference is harder to take and stay with than the negative; and when it is sexual, too, it demands much courage, honesty and respect from us in our countertransference responses."

(Alvarez, 2012, p. 129)

Notes

1 I searched Pep-Web and found 1,785 references for 'erotic transference' 592 references for 'erotic countertransference', 15 references for 'erotic transference, adolescence' and only 3 references for 'erotic countertransference, adolescence'. For a recent welcome exception see *Journal of Child Psychotherapy*, 2017, 43(1), in which the first three papers consider erotic transference within adolescent treatments. The editors comment that 'the literature on the topic has historically been somewhat slender' (Stratton and Russell, 2017).

2 For an exception to this generalisation, see Alvarez's description of "perverse sexuality" (Alvarez, 2012, p. 122) in a seven-year-old child.

3 It would be interesting to study the responses of adolescents to the use of the couch. In my experience some adolescents find the use of the couch sexually stimulating and some find it a refuge that helps them to talk about sexual feelings without having to look at the analyst, or either may be true at different times.

4 Person's (1985) paper on erotic transference in adults contends that male patients are more resistant to the awareness of the erotic transference and female patients are more resistant to the resolution of erotic transference in the cross-gendered treatments she studied. It would be interesting to study this question in adolescent treatments. In adolescence, particularly at puberty, the gender of the pair may matter more than at any other age.

5 In contrast to a classical view of countertransference as a hindrance, espoused by Reich (1951).

6 It is interesting to note the different but perhaps related issues that led this teen and his mother to accept a recommendation for more intensive work. Frank's acceptance of the recommendation followed his recognition of newfound vigour as he began to use his mind to separate himself from his mother's depression. His mother's not unrealistic concern that Frank would get in trouble with his risk-taking friends involved the dangers of separation.

7 Atkinson and Gabbard (1995) note that voyeuristic looking precedes genital sexuality in the ordinary sexual development of boys. Lena comments on a 16-year-old boy's gaze 'to penetrate into my eyes or to stare at my body. I felt very uncomfortable, embarrassed, intruded upon, at times repulsed by him' (Lena, 2016: 47). The intrusive quality of that boy's gaze was later understood as related to intrusion he had suffered. Frank's gaze seemed more as Atkinson and Gabbard describe.

8 See Laufer (1968: 115) re masturbation and masturbation fantasies in adolescence as 'trial actio' sometimes leading to developmental progression and sometimes to deadlock. My emphasis here is on the emergence of erotic feelings within the analytic work.

9 It is noteworthy that in the few articles I could find on erotic transference with adolescents, supervision was frequently mentioned: e.g. Lena: "Supervision represented a vital 'third' that enabled me to think about the dangers of focusing only on the maternal and infantile aspects while avoiding talking about sexuality ..." (Lena, 2017: 53).

10 Clearly Elise recognizes that "the analyst's creative energies are not to be a substitute for the absence of such energies in the patient; rather, they are best seen as an enlivening contribution to the analytic encounter, even if, paradoxically, they are used to narrate deadness and devitalization" (Elise, 2017: 51).

11 Anna Freud (1958) thought that adolescents separating from their objects were not able to sufficiently 'transfer' or attach to a new object, which made them difficult or impossible to treat. She felt that help might instead be aimed at their parents. Though many analysts did not share her view, it did seem to have a chilling effect on attitudes toward the intensive treatment of adolescents. A rare panel discussion at the American Psychoanalytic Association on analysis of adolescents, summarized by Sklansky, concluded 'few contemporary adolescent patients are analyzable... once in analysis a variety of parameters of technique far beyond those used in the classical analysis of adults are necessary' (Sklansky, 1972: 134). The one dissenting panellist was Adatto, who commented that certain adolescents with 'sufficient ego capacities and transference readiness can catapult an analysis into intensive productive work, rarely observed in adults' (ibid.: 138). More recent literature has emerged which differs from this concern regarding adolescent analysability (Laufer, 1997; Paz and Olmoz de Paz, 1992).

References

Alvarez, A. (2012). Types of sexual transference and countertransference in work with children and adolescents. In: *The Thinking Heart: Three Levels of Psychoanalytic Therapy with Disturbed Children*. Hove, East Sussex and New York: Routledge.

Anderson, R. (2004). *Adolescence and the body ego: The re-encountering of primitive mental functioning in adolescent development*. Unpublished paper presented at the 16th Annual Melanie Klein Memorial Lectureship, 8 January 2005, Los Angeles, CA.

Atkinson, S., and Gabbard, G. (1995). Erotic transference in the male adolescent-female analyst dyad. *Psychoanalytic Study of the Child* 50: 171–186.

Baranger, M. & Baranger, W. (2008). The analytic situation as a dynamic field. *International Journal of Psychoanalysis* 89: 795–826.

Bion, W.R. (1962). *Learning from Experience*. London: Heinemann.

Blum, H. (1973). The concept of the erotized transference. *Journal of the American Psychoanalytic Association* 21: 61–76.

Brady, M.T. (2016). *The Body in Adolescence: Psychic Isolation and Physical Symptoms*. New York: Routledge.

Davies, J.M. (1998). Between the disclosure and foreclosure of erotic transference and countertransference: can psychoanalysis find a place for adult sexuality? *Psychoanalytic Dialogues* 8: 747–766.

Dimen, M. (2011). *Lapsus linguae*, or a slip of the tongue: A sexual boundary violation in an analytic treatment and its personal and theoretical aftermath. *Contemporary Psychoanalysis* 47: 35–79.

Elise, D. (2017). Moving from within the maternal: the choreography of analytic eroticism. *Journal of the American Psychoanalytic Association* 65(1): 33–60.

Ferrari, A.B. (2004). *From the Eclipse of the Body to the Dawn of Thought*. London: Free Association Books.

Ferro, A. (1999). *The Bi-Personal Field: Experiences in Child Analysis*. London: Routledge.

Freud, A. (1958). Adolescence. *Psychoanalytic Study of the Child* 13: 55–278.

Freud, S. (1915). Observations on Transference Love. *S.E.* XII. London: Hogarth Press, pp. 159–171.

Greenberg, J. & Mitchell, S. (1983). *Object Relations in Psychoanalytic Theory*. Cambridge, MA: Harvard University Press.

Hartmann, S. (2017). Muriel Dimen, Field Theorist. *Studies in Gender and Sexuality* 18: 132–135.

Holtzman, D. & Kulish, N. (1997). *Nevermore: The Hymen and the Loss of Virginity*. Northvale, NJ: Jason Aronson Inc.

Jackson, E. (2017). Too close for comfort: the challenges of engaging with sexuality in work with adolescents. *Journal of Child Psychotherapy* 43(1): 6–22.

Kristeva, J. (2014). Reliance, or maternal eroticism. *Journal of the American Psychoanalytic Association* 62: 69–85.

Kulish, N. (1998). First loves and prime adventures: Adolescent expressions in adult analyses. *Psychoanalytic Quarterly* 67(4): 539–565.

Langs, R. (1981). *The Therapeutic Experience and its Setting*. New York: Jason Aronson Inc.

Laufer, M. (1968). The body image, the function of masturbation, and adolescence – problems of the ownership of the body. *Psychoanalytic Study of the Child* 23: 114–137.

Laufer, M. (1997). Developmental breakdown in adolescence: Problems of understanding and helping. In: Laufer, M. (ed.), *Adolescent Breakdown and Beyond*. London: Routledge.

Lena, F.E. (2017). Working with and "seeing through": sexual transference in the psychotherapy of an adolescent boy. *Journal of Child Psychotherapy* 43(1): 40–54.

Little, M. (1951). Counter-transference and the patient's response to it. *International Journal of Psychoanalysis* 32: 32–40.

Lombardi, R. (2016). *Entering one's own life as a goal of clinical analysis*. Unpublished paper presented at the Scientific Meeting, 14 November 2016, San Francisco Center for Psychoanalysis, San Francisco, California.

Lombardi, R. (2017). Body and mind in adolescence. In *Body-Mind Dissociation in Psychoanalysis: Developments after Bion*. London and New York: Routledge.

Molinari, E. (2017). *Field Theory in Child and Adolescent Psychoanalysis: Understanding and Reacting to Unexpected Developments*. London and New York: Routledge.

Ogden, T.H. (1994). The analytic third: working with intersubjective clinical facts. *International Journal of Psychoanalysis* 75: 3–19.

Ogden, T.H. (1995). Analyzing forms of aliveness and deadness of the transference-countertransference. *International Journal of Psychoanalysis* 76: 695–709.

Ogden, T.H. (1997). *Reverie and Interpretation*. Northvale, NJ: Jason Aronson Inc.

Paz, C. & Olmoz de Paz, T. (1992). Adolescence and borderline pathology: Characteristics of the relevant psychoanalytic process. *International Journal of Psychoanalysis* 73 (4): 739–755.

Paton, I. (2017). Within or without: negotiating psychic space with an adolescent at risk of developing a narcissistic personality structure. *Journal of Child Psychotherapy* 43(1): 23–39.

Person, E. (1985). The erotic transference in women and in men: differences and consequences. *Journal of the American Academy of Psychoanalysis and Psychiatry* 13: 159–180.

Racker, H. (1953). A contribution to the problem of counter-transference. *International Journal of Psychoanalysis* 34: 313–324.

Racker, H. (1957). The meanings and uses of countertransference. *Psychoanalytic Quarterly* 41: 303–357.

Reich, A. (1951). On countertransference. *International Journal of Psychoanalysis* 32: 25–31.

Samuels, A. (2000). The erotic leader. *Psychoanalytic Dialogues* 10: 277–280.

Searles, H. (1959). Oedipal love in the countertransference. *International Journal of Psychoanalysis* 40: 180–190.

Sklansky, M. (1972). Indications and contraindications for the psychoanalysis of the adolescent. *Journal of the American Psychoanalytic Association* 20(1): 134–144.

Stratton, K. & Russell, J. (2017) Editorial. *Journal of Child Psychotherapy* 43(1): 1–5.

Winnicott, D.W. (1949). Hate in the countertransference. *International Journal of Psychoanalysis* 30: 69–74.

Winnicott, D.W. (1971). *Playing and Reality*. London: Tavistock Publications.

8 In praise of modesty – in defence of a certain mystery

Ruggero Levy

Introduction

I would like to begin with a 16-year-old patient's description of a dream:

> I was in the *Grand Theft Auto* game. I thought how cool, here I can do anything I want. I got in my car; it had no door and was already beaten up from other adventures. I set off and saw three women in the street. I decided to "pick them up." I went up to the first one from behind, kissed her neck, but she turned around and attacked me. I got to the second one, put my hand on her ass and she got pissed off, too. Then I was in their car. The first two in the front and me with the third in the back. I started to "beat" her; she didn't want me to but she let me. But at some point she got up, stood up, said she was going to cum and peed on me. I didn't think it was bad. But then I masturbated and when I was going to cum, I came on her face. I thought, "Well done, you whore."
>
> Then I got out of the car, taking her phone, just to bother her. She came after me, asking for it back, but I got in my car and sped away, just for kicks. As it was in the game, she ran as fast as the car, beside the door, but the phone was on the other side and she had no way of reaching it. I kept laughing. But when I went to make a turn, the phone slipped and I saw it was going to fall. I thought, shit, she's going to catch it. So I said: "Take your fucking phone, I don't even want it." But when it fell out of the car, it exploded. I thought it was wonderful, because she looked like an idiot.
>
> I got out of the car and walked down the street in the middle of a lot of people. The women came after me, shouting at the others to catch me, that I was a bastard, but nobody did anything, I just laughed and thought that that was how it was because I could do anything in the game.

I will comment on this dream at the end of this paper.

André Green (1990) writes that psychism should be understood as an intermediary formation in the dialogue between the body and the world,

DOI: 10.4324/9781003380283-8

because this dialog is brutal, because the world's light is blinding and the body's demands tyrannical, and if we did not have this shock-absorbing formation formed by the conscious and unconscious psychism, we would still be in a pre-hominin stage.

(Green, 1990, p. 59)

That is, the subject is constituted in this dialogue between body and world, in the drive/object/culture interrelation. We should think like Cassirer (1997 p. 50) when he says that man should not be called *"animale rationale,"* but *"animale symbolocum"*, because man is an essentially symbolic being and this intermediate formation called psychism results from the symbolic transformations of our emotional experiences with others, our drives, desires and emotions.

The focus of my work lies in the idea that if symbolic processes are compromised, so too is the formation of the subject's whole subjectivity.

In 2023, how is the formation of human subjectivity constituted in the contemporary world after so many cultural changes? And contemporary psychoanalytic clinical practice? And the contemporary subject? And the contemporary adolescent?

As for the title, "In praise of modesty – in defence of a certain mystery", please do not be scandalized. In this chapter, I am not advocating a return to a retrograde sexual morality, prior to the sexual revolution of 1968. Rather, I am proposing a reflection on current times, using various reference points, to arrive at a psychoanalytical understanding of how this reality impacts the contemporary subject's mental functioning. Part of the title, is inspired by Alain Finkielkraut, a French philosopher who analyzed what he called the "New Love Disorder" (Lancelin, 2008). An old edition of the magazine *Le Nouvel Observateur* (Lancelin, 2008) studied the new sexuality of the French, based on extensive research conducted in France. It found what we can now also observe in Brazil: widespread contraception and, therefore, sexual freedom for women; the right to pleasure; the explosion of the couple as a stable structure; the emancipation of women in many aspects and areas of public life; recognition and greater acceptance of homosexuality; and the trivialization of pornography.

These are phenomenological findings that we need to understand from a metapsychological perspective. To grasp the contemporary phenomenon, in addition to understanding cultural changes and the revolution in sexual morals, we also need to comprehend the consequences of scientific and technological advances at a speed unprecedented in human history.

Since the second half of the 20th century, science has created new paradigms that have revolutionized the scenario of scientific thought and culture. New computer technology, from the sociological point of view (Bauman, 2000), has created a reality that generates a totally new feeling of insecurity and precariousness. But from the point of view of the subjectivation process, it has also created new phenomena in the field of symbolization (Levy, 2000). I refer to this in the second part of the title, "In defence of a certain mystery", inspired by Meltzer (1995). In his important contribution to the aesthetic conflict, Meltzer emphasizes the importance of the inaccessibility of the object's interior as a powerful stimulus to the imagination. The mystery of the intangible interior needs to be constructed by the creative imagination.

The question remains whether, with the overstimulation of the sensory by image culture, the loss of boundaries between the public and the private, and excessive exposure to nudity, to sexuality equated with pornography, the creative imagination and therefore human subjectivity may be compromised, and whether this leads to disturbances in the realm of desire and pleasure. I intend to develop the idea that the current culture promotes disturbances in the symbolic processes that can lead to damage in the construction of subjectivity.

In addition to the elements mentioned above, other characteristics of the contemporary, post-modern subject must be considered. This subject emerges from the complex integration between the digital world, globalization, hyper-consumerist society, and socio-economic reality, sharing some of their characteristics, as I will try to show.

I want to stress that I understand the subjectivity of the human subject as a property that emerges from a complex interaction between the individual's biology, the object relations where the individual developed, and the cultural context of their time.

But I propose that we consider the subject as follows: in all eras, we will come across cultural forces that promote symbolic processes, that is, of the expansion of the mind; and others that lead to the stagnation of psychic growth, sometimes to symbolic impoverishment, or even compromise to the symbolic function, constituting "dementalizing" forces that consequently open the way to passages to the act.

Psychoanalysis and subjectivation processes

Freud's great theoretical leap (1905) was to understand that human sexuality acquires its own autonomy supported by self-preservation drives. Thus, zones originally intended to satisfy vital functions acquire an erogeneity that then seek their own forms of pleasure and satisfaction. Sexual desire is constituted in the representation of these primitive experiences of satisfaction, and incessantly seeks its own satisfaction. Desire, then, is essentially a psychic motion (Laplanche, 1982) that will give the meaning of the object search (Kristeva, 1993) and of the unconscious fantasy. The dynamic force of the drive, transformed into desire, goes in search of the original object, which can never be found again. Thus, the corporal and the psychic are connected.

In this frame of reference, it is on repression, that is, from the constitution of symbolic substitutes of the desired object and the possibility of postponing immediate satisfaction, that the unconscious and the pre-conscious are structured with their extensive symbolic network. This constant pressure from within, under good symbolization conditions, will constantly change, expanding the mind infinitely. Seen from this theoretical perspective, this is how this symbolic network, our psychism and our subjectivity are constituted.

Green (1990) says that the system of mental representations that constitute our psychism, our "psychic life," is stimulated twofold: from the inside, by the transmutations of desire described above; and from the outside, by the excitation that is provoked on the pre-conscious/unconscious system. Bion and Meltzer studied how the encounter/disencounter with the object works as a powerful stimulus for the creation and expansion of our mental life. The great theoretical leap in Bionian contributions, developed by Meltzer, was to formulate that the presence of the object arouses a particular desire, the desire to know. Bion (1962) elevated the desire to know to almost the status of a drive.

In his theory of thinking, he established that when the mind is driven by the desire to know, it has a permanent symbolizing function that seeks to create for itself symbolic representations, versions, of the emotional experiences with which it is confronted. Perhaps as well as speaking of desire originating in the drive and primitive gratification experiences, based on Bion's contributions, we can speak of emotions that are at the core of the subject's experience. Of course, those emotions are triggered by desire, but also by the aesthetic impact of the external beauty of the object and the mystery of its interior, as described in *The Apprehension of Beauty* (Meltzer, 1995). It is evident how much the psychic life, the mind, is built from a subjective bond between subject and object and that the centre of this search is the subject's emotional experience, so to speak.

Meltzer (1995) also stressed the importance of the object's presence in the development of the mind and symbolization. Following Bion and understanding that the creative capacity occurs as a consequence of emotional experiences arising from the encounter with the object, he distinguishes between two types of relations in which human life is lived: those in which emotional experiences occur, and those in which they do not. He differentiates between two areas of human experience. There is an area of life and development that is dementalized and resembles the stimuli received by young animals, where learning through training, mimicry and conditioning predominates. This is the area marked by the presence of signs and conventions, rather than by the symbols themselves. It is an essential area for survival, similar to what Winnicott (1982) described as the false self. But it is expected that the human being will develop an area in which intimate relationships charged with emotional experiences can be established and learned about through thinking, so that from this, the imagination can build an image of the world (Meltzer, 1995).

In discussing the subject and its desire, we cannot overlook Winnicott's seminal contributions. In Winnicott's theory the baby has a desire and the good mother, in a state he calls primary maternal concern, presents and places the object of desire at the appropriate time and place. In doing so, she realizes the baby's omnipotence and gives it meaning; it is through the mother's strength and presence that the true self comes alive. The mother who is not good enough becomes centred in her ow desire, puts her gesture in the place of the baby's and the latter, in order to survive, submits to it, giving rise to the false self as a pathology of character.

Thus, it would be false to submit to a desire that is not one's own and adopt it as one's own. This happens when the relationship with an insufficiently good object – or culture – alienates the subject from their desire, from their emotions. For the purposes of this paper, I want to emphasize that the true self only acquires a living reality through the presence of the other that recognizes its desire. Again, this interests us, because we will see later how much our culture can lead the subject to be alienated from its own desire, either through disturbances in human and family bonds that we have observed, or through an excess of powerful stimuli that impose behaviours on the subject.

I would like to introduce here some of Bion's ideas (1962) about the possibility of enjoying the experience of satisfaction, since this leads to the idea that pleasure can exist without satisfaction. Kristeva (1993) talks about this when she says that contemporary humans, when they are not depressed, get excited about minor and devalued objects, in a perverse pleasure that knows no satisfaction (p. 14). But to return to Bion, in *Learning from Experience*, he says that there are situations in which the baby, out of his own or others' fear of certain emotions (e.g., hatred, envy, gratitude, etc.), refuses to drink the milk that the breast offers him. However, the baby realizes that he will then die. According to Bion, the baby, out of fear of death, resumes sucking from a deep dissociation in his mind. He starts to drink milk so as not to die, but this experience of material, bodily satisfaction is dissociated from psychic satisfaction. The baby solves the problem by destroying the ⊠ function.

Bion continues:

> This split [...] produces a mental state in which the patient greedily pursues every form of material comfort; he is at once insatiable and implacable in his pursuit of satiation. Since this state originates in a need to be rid of the emotional complications of an awareness of life, and a relationship with live objects, the patient seems to be incapable of gratitude or concern either for himself or others.
>
> (Bion, 1962)

What Bion describes is of the utmost importance. He describes a situation in which, due to fear of some emotions, there is an attack on the function, that is, the emotional experience of satisfaction cannot be transformed into elements, oneiric thoughts, and then understood through the gain of meaning from its mentalization, from its insertion into the reticle. In *Cogitations* (Bion, 1992, p. 223), Bion takes up the subject again, saying that when there is deficiency of the function the patient may even have a conscious, but cannot "become" conscious of certain emotional experiences, because he cannot "digest" them.

These experiences remain as "undigested facts," and only lend themselves to evacuation through the ⊠-screen.

In other words, when there is a disturbance of the symbolic processes, for whatever reason, despite material or bodily satiety, the subject remains mentally insatiable. An impossibility of experiencing psychic satisfaction is created, and dissatisfaction, hatred, remain as things in themselves, ⊠ elements that only lend themselves to being evacuated. The patient's objects become receptacles of his dissatisfaction.

When the ⊠-function, responsible for symbolization processes, is attacked, the subject's experiences become dementalized (Meltzer, 1990) in the protomental system, in which life is limited to an operative, almost mechanical, robotic functioning, and the subject is incapable of apprehending and enjoying the emotional meaning of his experience. Here lies the importance of understanding that failure or impairment in symbolic processes condemns the impossibility of satisfaction and, therefore, compulsive acting.

Returning to the origin of psychoanalysis, it was created on the understanding of the vicissitudes of desire. Freud understood that the neurotic symptom is established on the basis of repression and revolutionized the thinking of his time by challenging the culture of repression.

But human sexuality changes and metamorphoses constantly through time and culture. The drive as its strength and dynamics constantly seeks its own ways to satisfy itself. Today's culture has little to do with the Western European culture of the beginning of the last century. How to insert, then, sexuality, desire, pleasure and psychoanalysis in the present time?

Culture of uncertainty, simulation and performance

Several authors (Bauman, 1997; 2000; Cahn, 1999; Moreno, 2004; Eizirik, 2004; Menezes, 2004; Kristeva, 1993) have highlighted a new malaise present in modern culture: precariousness. Bauman (2000) states that "precariousness is everywhere today." Precariousness, vulnerability, and instability summarize contemporary life, in contrast with the stability, predictability, and consistency as a possible goal of modernity, the culture in which Freud worked. French theorists speak of *precarité*, the Italians of *incertezza*, the English of insecurity. All these concepts seek to grasp the phenomenon of the lack of guarantees and of instability in contemporary life.

I want to put forward that although I continue to analyze some characteristics of contemporary culture, we should not idealize modernity, since with its stability and search for rigid structures it also created "discontents," as Freud (1930) so masterfully wrote. The repudiation of the sexual in the 19th and early 20th centuries generated the great neuroses studied by Freud, with all that these represent in terms of obstacles to mental growth, and in doing so Freud challenged and confronted the culture of repression. The repudiation of the symbolic in contemporary culture is a great challenge for psychoanalysis today.

But to return to the precariousness of our cultural context, the unprecedented advance of technology in human history has created new illusions. Long-term insecurity makes instant gratification seem like a good deal, but in fact it is a trap. Everything in life has to be in the here and now. The postponement of satisfying desire has lost its fascination. Intolerance to frustration prevails. We know how important the postponement of satisfying desire is for the development of symbolic processes and, consequently, learning. It is in the space between desire and its fulfilment that thought is created. The present prioritization of immediate gratification, where historicization and deferral to the future make way, certainly affects the development of the creative imagination and the consequent expansion of the mental space necessary for the inscription of conflicts in the territory of the mental and their creation. In my opinion, this is one of the factors of contemporary life that affects symbolic processes, constituting a failure to favour the insertion, transmutation or resolution of conflicts linked to desire in the psychic realm. This is the moment when the symbolic networks essential to all subsequent development are built, not to mention the near abolition of latency in contemporary life (Guignard, 2005).

The fleeting nature of fashions and consumer objects creates a view of the world as "a container full of disposable objects, objects for one-off use – the whole world, including other human beings!" (Bauman, 2000, p. 186). The human bond becomes like any other consumer object, something that is expected to be immediately and instantly satisfied and that is rejected if it is not, creating a transience and instability in bonds, generating a new malaise in the culture, different from Freud's, resulting from sexual repression (Bauman, 1997).

To the fluidity of relationships is added the substitution of human bonds with virtual ones in which subjects, adolescents or otherwise, are isolated and solitary and take refuge in virtual relationships or in relationships that we could call narcissistic or utilitarian: the other is of interest as long as he or she satisfies my needs.

If we consider, like Meltzer, that it is in intimate relationships, charged with passion, that emotional experiences are created, and if we believe that these are what stimulate the mind to symbolization and its expansion, to growth, then we must admit that the immersion of the subject in a mechanical world introduces the subject into a universe where signs predominate, as a mechanical language to be dominated. Thus, it seems to me that the deep dive into the virtual world is yet another element of contemporary life that compromises the process of subjectivation. Besides favouring contacts of a narcissistic nature, it is a trivialization and an unprecedented accessibility to the world of perversion. In the same way, in this plunge into the world of virtual objects we do not have the presence of the object, with its gaze and its subjectivity giving reality to the subject's subjectivity, as Winnicott advocated.

The anti-imaginative activity of the image culture that Baudrillard mentions (1999) imposes itself strongly on the terrain of sexuality today. Young people no longer need to imagine the object of desire in order to masturbate. With one click, hyper real simulacra are in their room. A profusion of pornoerotic objects is at our disposal, or peers exposing themselves on webcams. The boundaries between public and private, between the erotic and the pornographic, are abolished, and, ultimately the imagination succumbs.

In this sense I agree with Menezes (2004, p. 85) when he says that in a time "without any sexual repression, with an unrestricted supply of sex, we see that the sexual succumbs". That is, the psychosexual originating in the unconscious, the fruit of transmutations of desire, succumbs to a sexual imposed by the culture of consumption, conveyed by celebrities in reality shows. It is a simulation of sexuality. This is the empire of the false self in which the subject is driven by a desire that is not their own. The subject adapts to a sexuality "as if," like other fashionable objects that must be adopted.

Kristeva (1993) says that contemporary humans have neither the time nor the space to constitute the soul, the mental; and the sexual that does not pass through symbolic elaboration becomes pleasure without satisfaction. This is pure discharge condemned to addictive compulsion by the impossibility of satisfying desire in the mental realm, much less its creation, as we shall see in the clinical case below.

Meltzer (1978) says that we have undergone a shift from the hypocrisy of the Victorian era to the hypocrisy of decadence. The cultural environment that once favoured the formation of symptoms in the realm of sexual conflict now favours the entrenchment of perversion in character. Culture often offers perverse paths to conflicts that were once constructed, undergone, and created – or not – on a symbolic level. The passage to the act is exalted as a solution to psychic suffering.

Another factor pushing for "dementalization" through the destruction of the meaning of emotional experience is the pressure for the medicalization of emotion (Rocha Barros, 2003). Physicians – and, by extension, psychoanalysts – are under pressure to eliminate any emotion slightly outside protocols established by pharmaceutical laboratories, regardless of meaning. Psychic pain and mental suffering need to be eliminated as soon as possible (Rocha Barros, 2003). I understand that this stimulus to the evacuation of psychic pain leads not only to the medicalization of emotion, but also to the mass use of legal and illegal drugs – the plague of post-modernity – and also to compulsive sexuality, whether promiscuous or not. The trivialization of perversion, the stimulus to eliminate psychic pain and to act upon it, often leads to the "solution" of conflicts through the creation of perverse sexual scenes. This addictive behaviour is stimulated by culture, and what becomes desired is euphoria and psychic anaesthesia (Ahumada, 2003). As Rocha Barros (2003) points out, euphoria becomes the model of "happiness." We find ourselves, thus, in the territory of pleasure without satisfaction, without satiety. In so far as it is not inscribed in the psychic as an experience of satisfaction, the compulsive need for the object of pleasure is created (drugs, material consumption, or sex as a drug). This is the culture of the simulation: euphoria equated with happiness; "having" equated with "being"; fetish and drug equated with the object; psychic anaesthesia equated with tranquillity.

More recently, Byung-Chul Han (2019) has made important contributions to the understanding of the postmodern performance subject, claiming that from the prevailing relations of productions, one launches into a performance project that gradually consumes one completely, although it is associated with a feeling – an illusion – of freedom. The demand for performance, self-imposed but coming from the performance culture of the system, makes the subject exploit himself beyond the real exploitations existing in the system. But the important consequence is that "the postmodern performance subject exploits himself until he becomes totally consumed (burnout), and then there is the emergence of self-aggressiveness that intensifies and not infrequently leads to suicide" (p. 25). And here we have the great invisible violence of today. What appears is its final result, the exhaustion or even the death of the subject. Han's theory is entirely compatible with the reality we are living where depression and suicide are reaching worrying levels, even before the COVID-19 pandemic. According to the WHO, diagnosed depression affects 4.4 per cent of the world population, 5.8 per cent in Brazil. Suicide figures are even more alarming, around 800,000 people worldwide take their lives each year. In Brazil, there are more than 12,000 suicides per year, and most shocking is that the vast majority are among young people aged between 10 and 29. In this range, the increase was 65 per cent between 10 and 14 years and 45 per cent between 15 and 19 years! Could this be due to the lack of opportunities and perspectives in a society where high performance and consumption are so highly valued?

Unlike the subject in modernity, where duty was the dominant element, the post-modern subject, inserted in the production system, mainly middle and upper class, aims not so much at obedience but at freedom and pleasure. Above all, the subject expects to derive pleasure from his work and listens mostly to himself and not to others (Han, 2019). However, freeing oneself from the other throws the performance subject into a relationship with himself, locking him in a narcissistic circuit, which is responsible for numerous psychic disturbances. This closing in on oneself, according to Han, causes a crisis of gratification, since it is not possible to gratify oneself insofar as recognition and gratification always occur in the relationship with the other, as we know from Freud's early contributions, but especially after Bion and Winnicott, who studied human development from an intersubjective perspective.

Due to the disturbance of the gratification structure, the performance subject finds himself forced to produce and perform more and more until he reaches burnout or depression, according to Han, if not suicide. "The narcissistic plunge into the self does not generate gratification, but instead imposes pain on the self" (p. 62). As I said before, this system of self-exploitation constitutes one of today's great invisible forms of violence.

Very close to Bion's ideas, Han states, "when experiences are made, we encounter the other; experiences alter us" (p. 63). Like Winnicott, Han states that if the relationship with the other is totally lost, one cannot form a stable self-image (p. 63).

While Byung-Chul Han seems to know Freud's works well, he restricts psychoanalysis to them. Hence he claims that psychoanalysis can only understand the subject of modernity, which he calls the subject of obedience. He says that this subject is the subject of negativity insofar as repression; the impossibility of gratifying the drive, is what causes neurosis. The impossibility of expressing and gratifying the drive causes the illness of the subject of obedience. However, he argues that since the performance subject is post-modern, the subject of positivity, of excess, is outside Freudian understanding. This statement is partially true, since Freud indeed supported his understanding of neuroses based on the mechanism of repression, even when referring to current neuroses, guided by an excess of anxiety not linked to representations resulting from an excessive repression.

However, Han seems to ignore the post-Freudian contributions of Bion, Winnicott, Green and Roussillon, who understand that psychism is structured in an intersubjective dimension, from the encounter with the other and the mind, through symbolization processes, with the task of containing, transforming and representing the stimuli and emotions arising from the body or from the encounter with the other and the world.

From these contributions, one can understand the functioning of the so-called performance subject exposed to a number of frustrations arising from an infinite and unattainable demand for performance, whether in the realm of the professional, sexual, or bodily care. An excess of frustrating sensations and emotions is created that overwhelm the capacity for representation and end up being traumatic, leading to burnout and depression, afflictions that are highly prevalent in our time. And here we see a compromise in the formation of subjectivity, insofar as there are a number of unrepresented emotions that lead to prevalent clinical symptoms besides depression and burnout, such as drug addictions, psychosomatic diseases, anorexia, bulimia, etc.

In this sense, Han states "The process of repression or negation plays no role in contemporary psychic maladies such as depression, burnout, and ADHD. Instead, they indicate an excess of positivity [...] the inability to say no [...] being-able-to-do-everything" (Han, 2019, p. 67).

Final comments, or, in defence of mystery

Evidently, to the extent that we live in diverse microcultures, the whole spectrum of patients may visit our office, with the usual neurotic symptoms; those in whom the pathology is expressed in their behaviour and in their body by insufficiencies in symbolization processes; and also with what we could call neo-solutions to sexual conflict based on the adoption of paths offered by culture, guided by acting out, narcissism, and perversion.

Returning to the patient's dream, I described this material because it illustrates part of the cultural environment in which we live. The type of "solution" offered by culture in the face of frustration: the free land trumpeted by the video game is the place where freedom is equated with a lack of limits; where the subjectivity of others with their pains and desires does not matter, the subject is restricted to his narcissistic bubble; and one can give vent to one's desires omnipotently, whenever and however one wishes. In dreams, this world of pre-genital pleasures is symbolized oneirically. But, unfortunately, it is often acted out without the mediation of the symbolic, but with the mediation of legal and illegal drugs. Raves and parties fuelled by MDMA (methylenedioxy-methamphetamine, commonly known as ecstasy), in combination with other drugs, are perhaps the materialization of this world. At such parties, people seek a dementalized state that allows the acting out of this narcissistic universe with a perverse colouring. Evidently, this patient presented a personal psychopathology that included a difficulty in the construction of his masculine identity stemming from an identification with a fragile father involved in a parental relationship in which the mother was felt to be phallic. This was exhaustively analyzed in multiple possible aspects: in his fear and avoidance of women; in his fantasies and impotence; in his relations with his peer group, where initially he masochistically submitted to his friends; in the transference where I sometimes felt like a kind of "analyst/phallus" who knew everything and could do everything; and sometimes as someone who could be martyred.

However, much more than discussing the case of this patient, I wanted to illustrate how my patient's adolescent confusion in which an inadequate defensive split (Meltzer, 1998) of sexuality, with masculinity equated with violence, found ways to express itself, empowered by elements offered by culture. The cultural influence is much more pronounced with adolescents, precisely because they are rebuilding their system of representations, their subjectivity, as it offers, emphasizes or encourages certain forms of expression of sexuality.

I agree with Rocha Barros (2003) that in this terrain of "new forms of sexuality," psychoanalysis is also under great pressures, since the dividing line between what is normal and what we still find pathological is blurred, and not accepting certain sexual behaviours as normal seems to be a prejudiced, ideological and therefore unacceptable position.

> The analyst is pressured not to use his investigative spirit in relation to certain sexual transgressions and to consider them as normal. We then run the risk of losing the opportunity to distinguish between what could be a simple sexual option, of a pathological use of sexuality, transformed into a perversion of character, if we succumb to ideological pressure.
>
> (Rocha Barros, 2003, p. 5)

Evidently, the possibility of succumbing to these pressures is greater the more we lose belief in the theoretical-technical arsenal of psychoanalysis.

This insufficiency in symbolic processes that I have referred to throughout this chapter has had numerous consequences. First, as I explained, the difficulty of registering the experience of satisfaction in the psyche leads to an unsatisfied jouissance, to the repetition of the pulsional discharge in a compulsive way. Ahumada (2003) emphasizes that this compromising of the capacity to represent causes the primitive, non-elaborated psychic contents to surface increasingly. Acting out, violence, self-destructive behaviours, the sexual invaded by the destructive is highly present. This damage to the symbolic processes then leads to an unfinished process of subjectivation. This, in turn, pushes towards narcissistic pathologies that affect behaviour and the body, such as delinquency, anorexia, bulimia, massive drug use, depression and, not infrequently, suicide. Narcissistic defences seek to solve the insufficiency of psychic elaboration (Cahn, 1999).

This has direct implications for psychoanalytic technique. In addition to bearing the cultural pressure to immediately eliminate any psychic suffering, the mind of the analyst becomes of almost decisive importance, as it will often take an enormous amount of reverie work to create mentalizations out of raw sensations and emotions that patients bring with them. The development of mental space through the establishment of an intimate relationship in analysis becomes the priority and a challenge, as it goes against the pressures of the culture of narcissism. Finkielkraut (1988) defines well that we live in the culture of sensations and feeling as opposed to the word. So our goal is to turn sensations into symbols, thoughts, and then into words, since sensations are only to be felt, experienced, or acted upon.

Mental growth is only possible through the symbolic transformation of emotion experienced in an intimate relationship, and in this sense we have to understand this whole environment in which we are inserted, the difficulties in establishing deep human bonds and also the damage to the constitution of subjectivity due to symbolic failures. The challenges that we face range from representational emptiness to what I would call thoughts/pseudo-thoughts or conducts/prostheses; pseudo-thoughts or conducts grafted from culture that are used as prostheses to fill symbolic voids or used to replace the process of psychic elaboration.

I agree with Donaldo Schüler when he says that psychoanalysis is the reliquary of the word. This is the revolution that psychoanalysis needs to make at the dawn of the 21st century, to fight for the revival of interest in thinking and meaning in the warmth of human relationships guided by passion (Meltzer, 1990). So, if Freud challenged and faced the culture of repression with his rejection of the sexual, in today's culture we must challenge and face the rejection of the symbolic. This is the great challenge of psychoanalysis today. I think that every area of activity concerned with the human psyche has this responsibility to be the reliquary of the symbolic. And for this the mystery of the interior of the object, non-intrusiveness, respect for limits, is essential. Fortunately, we are not alone in this. There are countless other areas of culture and science that promote an increase in the capacity for abstraction, in the development of the human mind. To close, I give as an example an idea of Alain Finkielkraut, when he says that modesty is not just an archaic moralism, but an ontological attribute of women. Female sexuality implies the existence of something hidden, to be unveiled, or constructed by the imagination, some mystery. Excessive shamelessness, excessive light and exposure extinguishes the light of imagination. Hence, in praise of modesty and the defence of a certain mystery.

References

Ahumada, J. (2003) O inconsciente na pós-modernidade: as tensões epistêmicas. *Revista de Psicanálise da SPPA* 10(3): 495–507.

Baudrillard, J. (1999) *Tela total – mito-ironias da era do virtual e da imagem*. Porto Alegre: Editora Sulina.

Bauman, Z. (1997) *O Mal-estar na pós-modernidade*. Rio de Janeiro: Jorge Zahar.

Bauman, Z. (2000) *Modernidade líquida*. Rio de Janeiro: Jorge Zahar.

Bion, W. (1962) *Aprendiendo de la Experiência*. Mexico City: Paidós.

Bion, W. (1992) *Cogitations*. London: Karnac Books.

Cahn, R. (1999) *O adolescente na psicanálise – a aventura da subjetivação*. Rio de Janeiro: Companhia de Freud.

Cassirer, E. (1997[1944]) *Ensaio Sobre o Homem*. São Paulo: Martins Fontes.

Eizirik, C. (2004) Sexualidade e pós-modernidade. *Revista de psicanálise da Sociedade Psicanalítica de Porto Alegre* 11(1): 87.

Ferro, A. (1998) *Na sala de análise*. Rio de Janeiro: Imago.

Finkielkraut, A. (1989) A derrota do pensamento. São Paulo: Editora Paz e Terra.

Freud, S. (1905) Três Ensaios Sobre uma Teoria da Sexualidade. *ESB*, VII. Rio de Janeiro: Imago.

Freud, S. (1930) Mal Estar na Civilização. *ESB*, XXI. Rio de Janeiro: Imago.

Green, A. (1990) *Conferências brasileiras – Metapsicologia dos limites*. Rio de Janeiro: Imago.

Guignard, F. (2005) Psicanálise e sexualidade hoje. *Revista de psicanálise da SPPA* 12(2): 247–261.

Han, Byung-Chul (2019) *Topologia da violência*. Rio de Janeiro: Editora Vozes.

Kristeva, J. (1993) *As novas doenças da alma*. Rio de Janeiro: Rocco.

Lancelin, A. (2008) Eloge de la pudeur. In: *Le Nouvel Observateur*, Paris.

Laplanche, J. (1997) *Vocabulário de Psicanálise: Laplanche e Pontalis*, sob a direção de D. Lagache. São Paulo: Martins Fontes.

Levy, R. (2000) *Do símbolo à simbolização: uma revisão da evolução teoria e as repercussões sobre a técnica psicanalítica*. Trabalho para Membro Efetivo, presented at SPPA, January 2000.

Meltzer, D. (1973) *Os Estados Sexuais da Mente*. Rio de Janeiro: Imago.

Meltzer, D. (1978). *The Kleinian Development Part 1*. Perthshire: Clunie Press.

Meltzer, D. et al. (1990) *Metapsicologia Ampliada – aplicações clínicas dos conceitos de Bion*. Buenos Aires: Spatia Editorial.

Meltzer, D. (1995) *A Apreensão do Belo*. Rio de Janeiro: Imago Editora.

Meltzer, D. (1998) *Adolescentes*. Buenos Aires: Spatia.

Menezes, L.C. (2004) Sexualidade e pós-modernidade. *Revista de psicanálise da Socie-dade Psicanalítica de Porto Alegre* 11(1): 79.

Moreno, J. (2004) Sexualidade e pós-modernidade. *Revista de psicanálise da Sociedade Psicanalítica de Porto Alegre* 11(1): 69.

Rocha Barros, E. da (2003) *Pre-formed counter-transference: a response to the patient or to the culture?* Presented on the panel, Frontiers of Psychopathology: New Culture, New Patients, IPA Congress, Toronto.

Winnicott, D.W. (1982) Distorção do ego em termos de verdadeiro e falso self. In: *O ambiente e os processos de maturação*. Porto Alegre: Artes Médicas.

9 Towards the construction of the adult identity

Another adolescent mourning

Michele Ain

The construction of the adult identity

As the progressive abandonment of the adolescence takes place, the adult life begins, to which we can assign logical time, but not chronological time. Defining the end of adolescence is quite relative, even though in different premises seems like it is relevant to do so with certain precision: in biology, the academic, social, and legal fields. And it is from the social field where it seems to appear a greater need of categorizing and segmenting since they tend to define a certain lifestyle, which also entails peculiarities in consumption groups: X generation, Y generation, millennials, centennials …

The adult identity is constructed, it is not a pre-existing objective that has to be reached. Psychoanalysis – in its essence – addresses and deepens into the distinctive features of the subject, looking into the individual peripeteia, their history and their own process of subjectivation without subscribing to a rigid and standardized normative.

During adolescence, the identifying reorganization "threatens" the narcissistic bases for it brings with itself the dis-investiture of infantile objects. This will be a time of assembly between the body, the self-image and the ideals, in which the sexed body will have to be metaphorized. Naturally, this transit will not be free of emerging anguishes from the implied conflicts. The succession of griefs inherent to growing up will stage the conflictive dilemma between the wish to grow up and be independent and wanting to remain attached to the safety of the infantile dependence.

The consequential rearrangement of the place in the family, taking a position such as being sexed, along with achievements such as work integration, economic independence, reconciliation with the body and the assumption of new commitments and responsibilities, will bring along the gradual concretion of life projects. What a simple task… a trip from primary helplessness to insertion in a world that tends to the aspiration of a certain hollow omnipotence.

Emerging from the intricate bond between ideals (achieved to a greater or lesser extent) and identifying processes that settle – beyond its own dynamism – will forge the constitution of an identity and a character sufficiently

DOI: 10.4324/9781003380283-9

stable, that is able to allow psychic reorganization, after the difficult work of transiting through adolescence.

Identity encloses a paradox: it is a prior condition of the recognition and acceptance of the alterity, as well as being a guarantor of a reassuring preservation of subjectivity, abandoning the aspiration of an illusory ubiquity (Ladame, 1999).

After having reached certain identitarian cohesion and narcissistic affirmation, in times where the Ego will also organize itself around limits, defences and its vassalage, the subject will be ready to head towards the materialization of their projects and the fulfilment of their wishes with a certain leeway, because determinants of the personal, social and cultural context are unavoidable.

Is it, at the present time, harder for adolescents to achieve their ideals, reach their goals, more so than it was for the preceding generation? This has never been a simple task, and as the modern utopia seemed as if it could offer the possibility of distinguishing, almost without hesitation, the good from the bad, post-modern scepticism keeps us from the certainties in its function that it is the legitimate guarantor of a socially consensual value system.

We support a tendency towards loosening of family and social bonds, the exaltation of a wandering individualism, and the search for autonomy and independence to the detriment of the adoption of new and complex responsibilities.

Knowledge resides in Google and is not embodied in referential figures, which blurs the position of limits inherent in the adult world, that often gives in its function, lost in the social ideal of youth. This seems to carry new ways of searching for limits during adolescence: self-inflicted wounds, academic failure, social phobia, eating disorders, diverse addictive behaviours, configured as symptomatic forms of a request for help and boundaries.

We agree with the claim of the present as the only period, unified and of immediate obsolescence. The past is gone and the future is now. How have we, not so young adults, accommodated these changes in the subjectivity, to this "civilizing mutation"? (Viñar, 2000).

How, from the place of adulthood, do we promote or restrict exchange and relations with the new generations?

This is a huge challenge: maintaining our adult role, not fusing with, or mistakenly taking refuge in the lack of generational distance, not surrendering our function, without stopping a promotion of exchange, encounter and enrichment that the permeability in the approach with youth can allow.

Counter to what appears to be established, this requires us to change, to have the sufficient plasticity to abandon certain convictions that are rooted and functional to the times we were brought up in, and to find the necessary disposition to search, create and recreate tools to be in the world ... it was unforeseen.

We may think that in the history of culture, the conflicts of the human soul have been basically the same, but with the distance between generations that coexist today, they seem emphasized by the velocity of change, as well as increased life expectancy. Paradoxically, globalization and technological revolution favour a certain blurring between the generational differences, and constantly test us, in our clinical practice as well.

How does a teenager picture their future today, at a time where demand for success encompasses economic aspects to a certain ideal of excellence, and in which the concept of progress – more individual than social – seems to be a purpose in itself, more than a path to the accomplishment of personal or collective gratifications and aspirations of improvement?

Investing a project has as a precondition a recognition of the risk that will imply admitting and accepting the difference between reality and fantasy, acknowledging the distance between what is accomplished and what stays entrenched in ideals. It does not seem easy, if it ever has been, more so, in times that promote any avoidance of frustration and delayed gratification.

Possibly the hardest facts to metabolize are the apology of uncertainty, the pregnancy of the present that leaves the future in suspense, together with a generalized idealization of youth, that exhausts euphemisms in the desire to deny the passing of time, and death. Everything happens now, waiting is poorly tolerated, anxiety and velocity win, and the capacity for amusement seems to have lost its potential to surprise, and it seems like everything is already known before it is actually understood.

The Ego is being constructed, always in gerund, at the cost of the elaboration of multiple griefs and their traumatic effect, which will lead to changes in its constitution, in relation to the search for new objects (not incestuous) as well as the possibility of other sublimated libidinal investitures, guiding the path to the progressive detachment of parental and social aspirations, to find and give place to the subject's own. And it widens and becomes enriched when it finds the crack from where it listens to their own voice, different to the sole discourse (of parents/adults) of the infantile Superego.

In this way the difficult identification and dis-identification process offers the Ego a path, a knowledge about the future Ego, and a knowledge about the future of the Ego (Hornstein, 2015).

Leaving adolescence after a period that sometimes feels unproductive, or a time when nothing is accomplished, has buried an arduous unconscious psychic work in search of identity and recognition, and the encounter with the potentiality of projecting a possible future, an innovative "being in the world".

In psychoanalysis we have a certain tendency to consider adolescence only by emphasizing its turbulent, critical aspects and psychic reorganization during this period, with all that it implies, and that must be endured through to reach adulthood. We often forget that this is a process that never fully ends, and it continues to generate effects more or less silently. Similarly, before this critical and painful time, it tends to be underestimated what it means in terms of the novelty that is experimented, the large acquisitions and prerogatives that imply growing up and that gain structuring value.

In regard to the Oedipus Complex, André Green (1993) proposes that it does not become exhausted, neither does it disappear or become extinguished, but dissolves like salt in water, since its unconscious organizing effect of the psyche remains. We can make the same idea extend to adolescence, that it is not fully relieved by adult life, but also seems to be diluted like salt in water, and will come about, in the aprés-coup time, to be the paradigm of all mutative fantasies. Growing up, Green states, will inevitably "make us renounce to the satisfaction in which one is the jewel, the pearl, the pupil of the mother's eye".

Is one ever healed from that?

The clinic

Often when we work with patients, we are surprised that while they have accomplished a good transit through adolescence and the concretization of yearned and sought projects begins, a surprising anguish-stained crisis bursts, apparently inexplicably, since everything appears to be going along the expected track and sometimes exceeds individual, parental and social expectations.

These frequent poundings, apparently disruptive, evidence the necessity to elaborate a new grief, like a bump on a log: this time, for a lost adolescence, or what was lost during adolescence, that time now idealized as liberty, full of potential, of enjoyment of life with peers and continuous discovery of all kinds of acquisitions.

At other times, when childhood and the passage through adolescence has been very turbulent and troubled, and the parental bond fragile and inconsistent, the relatively solid identifications that organize an Ego that is cohesive, integrated, and able to resort to more elaborate defence mechanisms in which the symbolization offers greater elaborative possibilities, are not achieved. We observe great psychic fragility, with serious difficulties in metabolizing frustrations. Adulthood appears, in the image of Chronos, announcing that the time of the adolescence has passed, but leaving as evidence the defencelessness and difficulty in growing, sometimes hidden and effectively crouched beneath strong and costly defence mechanisms.

I will describe some clinical vignettes that even though they are, necessarily, short cuts, they will illustrate these vicissitudes.

Emilia, at 23 years old, finished her tertiary studies and began working in her profession very successfully, which allowed her to achieve independence, moving away from her parents' home and moving in with her boyfriend to a new place, after many years of having begun analysis.

She was achieving many, very yearned for projects. However, she started feeling, somewhat untimely, intense discomfort and anguish. She could not comprehend it … everything appeared to go as expected. She began to bring very prolific dreams to the sessions.

> Yesterday I could not stop crying. I went to my parents to visit, but I could not distract myself. I kept dreaming… I dreamt I went to the grocery store, but I was not there to pick anything up. I ate cake with some

children that were there and I tried to leave but I could not do so, and an alarm was going off.

She told me that ever since she had moved out, she dreamt of her mother a lot, of her scolding her as she helps her pick her clothes out and also of people that die … "It anguishes me to think that everything I do each day, someday will be just a memory". "I had a dream where I lost everything. I left everything on the bus, my purse, my documents, my phone … in a grocery store I found my ID. And with that, I was able to reconstruct everything else that was missing."

She dreams and puts into action her conflicts and wishes.

Going back to her parents in search of refuge and comfort stages what the dream reveals. Emilia does adult things, she works, is independent, goes to the grocery store, but the anguish sets her back to the infantile scene: she gets locked up with some children eating cake, at her parents' house, with her siblings? Returning to the loss of childhood and also trying, unsuccessfully, performing as an adult. The wish to go back to times where the mother tells the little girl off and helps her get dressed appears.

As, in the dream, she expresses the loss of "everything", the adult life confronts her with a renovated version of adolescent grief, grief for that period of time, and its circumstantial identity reorganization. In this way, this absolute "everything" accentuates the experience of danger of orphanhood, doubting her proven capacity to be an adult. Growing up, being an adult, was and is something she yearned for, charged with projects and motivations. However, she is surprised by the anguish that she is facing, which is also a longing for an idealized time where the dependency on endogamic figures were guarantors of her stability.

I dreamt that I came to the session, but it was somewhere else and an old friend of mine, named just like me, was also there. I did not know what to do, her and I sat at the divan. Somewhere in the middle there was a small table with a baby, healthy, a bit independent, wanting to walk. You said we should change the schedule of the session because it was difficult having to take care of that defenceless baby. In the middle, my father showed up and I got upset and made him leave. … Afterwards I went to have lunch at my parents' and wrote in my notebook: "It is not my home anymore, I am another daughter, the real one. My parents are also new. I am puzzled by myself, the past is the only place to go, the present is an obligated time …"

She dreams and writes, also about her dream.

How to be "someone else" without having to stop being herself?

Inside her, her current self and the defenceless baby that has to be taken care of, coexist. She is an adult and also a slightly independent baby, carrying great fear of living out her independence, which she also enjoys. I, as analyst, assist with the coexistence of her before and now, the one from the past and the "forced" present, and I seem to embody the limit – blurry, of course – that means to process the grief for the childhood, to be another one and the same, just like her parents, and that produces estrangement.

It is as if I were asked, who is this adult? And it seems to find the answer in that complex coexistence of the baby, her past self, and her current self, that evokes to me Russian dolls. And eventually, ejecting the father, who appears in a place where he does not belong, endorses that the decanting of the Oedipic aspirations does not switch them off. They are salt in water, and every once in a while, they resurge demanding greater psychic work.

How can we accept that the passing of time turns everything into a memory? Perhaps with the condition of accepting that memories are what remains of what is lost.

Ana is 20 years old. Her father passed away when the family lived abroad and she has lived with her mother since they returned to the country. The relationship between them is extremely conflictive and hostile. Ana studies at university and leads a life almost fully dedicated to confront and defend herself from the maternal battering. She recognizes herself as not very cared for, exposed, extorted and neglected throughout her upbringing. Adolescence exposed this impossibility of an encounter even further. She grew up very lonely at the expense of rigid and impassable defence mechanisms, because, as she told me, "it is a matter of survival". The exchange, interests, and the bond itself with her mother relies on basically giving her, or not giving her money or material things. Sometimes, the mother seems to want to reach out to her, but it always turns out to be unfruitful. She can withstand the limits that the alterity implies, consider her daughter as another desiring being, and oscillates between neglect and overwhelm.

This has brought, among other things, an intense transferential bond, in which the dependence and demands turn very intense, and that demands from me a special care, as well as a permanent questioning of my position-ing, oscillating between being there and supporting her – she needs it – as well as setting boundaries of the alterity and favouring her possibility of growth. A difficult analytic work that necessarily confronts the raw material reality with destructive fantasies and the libidinal aspirations that appear destined to a failure to encounter, and that our work tends to bind.

Ana is desperately looking to move out and stay away from such a destructive cohabitation. Her mother also approves but only passively assists to the possibility of achieving it. Ana, paradoxically, wishes for it, believes it is necessary, but does not feel ready.

In her, there is a coexistence of mature and critical aspects, she tries to plan her future but cannot resist the force that is keeping her next to her mother to continue to demand what she cannot give to her, and to reproach her what she did not have. In addition, there are very fragile and dependent aspects to her, with difficulty in the management of her autonomy as a result of her painful story: non-elaborated grief, a childhood with multiple estrangements underestimated by her environment, a lonely adolescence that never allowed her to consolidate her identity. Like this, oscillating between achieving personal aspirations and a greater autonomy, she confronts her defenceless side, a product of infantile neglect, which we are focusing on during the analysis. Past, present and future knotted in a difficult plot that we will have to continue to work on so that Ana can, yet not without hurdles, project an autonomous life.

Pedro is 21 years old. He began analysis, during the last year of tertiary studies which took place abroad, due to a serious anxiety disorder, and physical symptoms, particularly ahead of university exams. He has always been a very good student. During the holidays, he returned to the country to work in his father's business. He enthusiastically studies to take charge of the family business, a plan that has been established since Pedro can remember, and in which his father has set all expectations regarding him. And these are the only expectations. He does not know much about his son's life, his preoccupations and his personal life, since forever. He occasionally asks him about his grades. And Pedro gets angry and reproaches him for it, but his father does not seem to comprehend or be able to have another type of approach.

During the analysis, failure to meet with his father, his anguish, not conscious for Pedro, which implies satisfying the paternal expectancy that he has made his own, have led him in many aspects to live like an adult since his adolescence, has had a very relevant place. Let us listen to him: "My father is crazy. Everything people do, he thinks it is against him. I call him Carlos, that is his name, because he is not a father. Ever since I was 15 years old, he has taken me on holidays to work with him so that I can train for the job. Ok! Yes. I am interested, I love it. But I have not had a life as a young person, I never have … I look 30 since I have been 15! It is not fair. Help me, because I think I still have time … My friends always tease me with that matter. They call me Mister. And I tell them that they will shortly have to call me Master …"

Pedro has performed as an adult since he was very young. He had that place assigned and was seduced by the identification with a successful father that grants him succession, yet he has not been able to confront him. He also has not been able to listen to his own adolescent wishes and concerns. He could not find that crack through which he could question the life that had been imagined for him. Fortunately, Pedro, with his symptoms and his anxiety could tell that something was not right, he listened to the signals of his body, that became ill ahead of each test, and the overwhelming anxiety he experienced, talked about how conflictive and distressing it was to be himself, detaching himself from strong paternal expectations to find the breach that exists between what he can do and what the ideals impose. And this breach, finding himself, accepting the fact that he is human, that he can quit being everything that he is expected to be. Accepting that he can be himself, young, live the experiences that his parents lived, without feeling like he is failing in his adult aspects, knowing he can wish for something else, and expanding his critical view – which he has – to other fields of his life to be able to construct a proper identity, with which he feels consolidated. I also do not think it is about living the adolescence that he did not have. It would be very simplistic and would imply denying what could not be. It is about assembling now, in the aprés-coup time, the skipped, more infantile over-looked aspects, with the renewed expectancy that he can integrate them.

I still vividly remember the impression that produced reuniting with Clara at 23 years of age after finishing her analysis two years before. She calls me to ask for an interview. I recalled having said goodbye to her during the summer, some time before her graduation from Law University. She was wearing flat sandals, very juvenile clothes, it was the holiday season with her friends, her long hair covering her back. Now I see her arriving with her dejected face, her hair up, glasses, a purse and another bag for her work computer, a formal suit … and I thought I could intuit her before listening. She cried while she said:

> I cannot take it anymore. I want to quit. I got my degree, and I have been in this job for six months, which is pretty good, I like it, the pay is good. But I do not know why I cannot stand it anymore. I want to quit and my parents will not let me! Oh! And I also want to leave Lucas (her boyfriend).

The impact that her physical change caused accounted for what was happening.

Clara was impacted by seeing herself as an adult. She wanted to leave everything that reminded her of it. Adolescence with her friends at the beach had abruptly given way to this young adult who could not feel herself in that place. She was talented and a successful student. But she could not comfor-tably wear that suit. And she naturally accepted that her parents would not allow her to quit … We worked on this for a few months. Her difficulty in assuming adulthood, the fantasized solution of leaving all behind with the illusory idea of going back to being an adolescent, the weight – secondary benefit – of her parents' opinion, which incarnated some proper aspects, her impulse to the exogamic object. Finally, after encountering that pending grief for the lost adolescence, and being able to elaborate that anguish, she was able to successfully lead her adult life.

I mention it, because the image when I saw her again, which I remember so vividly, became paradigmatic for me, as a product of what it encapsulates, it shows what, to my understanding, happens many times with the assumption and the beginning of the adult life.

Becoming an adult is a new psychic work, bound to prehistory, history and the future of the subject, in times that will crimp and reaccommodate during life in new turns of the spiral. More than the finishing point of a better or worse transited adolescence, in terms of suffering and new acquisitions, and it will relaunch at the same time new challenges and experiences, adulthood constructs and can consolidate in the measure that it constitutes a tool to confront the autonomous life supported on the ability for critical thought.

Like so, Umberto Eco writes on a letter to his son:

> ... And tomorrow? What will happen to a childhood where during industrial Christmas brings American dolls that talk and sing, Japanese automatons that jump and dance? ... So, dear Stefano, I will gift you a rifle. And I will teach you to play in very complicated wars where one can never side with just one part ... You will vent ... In your young years you will confuse ideas a bit, but some convictions will slowly be born. Then, as an adult, you will believe that it was all a story, Little Red Riding Hood, Cinderella, the rifles, the cannons, the man against the man ... But if, by chance, when you are older, the monstrous figures of your childhood dreams still exist ... witches, armies, bombs, compulsory recruitment, I hope you have acquired a critical conscience towards fairy tales and you learn to move critically in reality.
>
> (Eco, 1964)

References

Eco, U. (1964). *Segundo Diario Mínimo*. Madrid: Lumen, p. 36.

Green, A. (1993). El adolescente en el adulto. *Revista por la Asociación Psicoanalítica de Buenos Aires* 15(1): 39–68.

Hornstein, L. (2015). *Adolescencias Contemporáneas*. Buenos Aires: Psicolibro.

Ladame, F. (1999). ¿Para qué una identidad? O el embrollo de las identificaciones y de su reorganización en la adolescencia. *Revue française de psychanalyse* 4: 405–415.

Viñar, M.N. (2000). El Psicoanálisis en el Vértigo de la Mutación Civilizatoria; la práctica psicoanalítica en el contexto actual. *Revista Uruguaya de Psicoanálisi* 91: 160–176.

10 Working with adolescents: formlessness, fears and transformation

Nergis Güleç

Adolescence and formlessness

If we define transformation roughly as giving a new shape or form to something original, perhaps we can think of adolescence as a period of a potential transformation process of formlessness or not – adolescents are no longer children yet they are not adults. They find their bodies so foreign, and feelings so inappropriate that perhaps we can define their situation as formless. It is as if everything felt to be known by the adolescent has changed: their psyche, body, and parental figures, their thoughts and beliefs have all become unfamiliar, and the general governing atmosphere seems to be uncanny. Even their tone of voice sounds different; their arms and legs move as if they don't belong to their body and their impulses drive them psychically from one place to another making them feel out of control.

Freud (1937) in "Analysis Terminable and Interminable", defines adolescence as the period where the pressure of the drives is of utmost intensity. While their relatives observe them disbelievingly, they too cannot understand what is going on inside themselves. Everything seems to have changed quantitatively (intensity) and qualitatively (content). Thus, with the addition of new feelings and experiences, all representations need to be re-evaluated and transformed. Adults, peers, groups, and sometimes art and literature, who do not retaliate, can all contribute to this transformation. In order to grow, some things need to be buried, killed, and left behind. What is left behind and killed symbolically during adolescence are parents, and childishness. But as this allows for growth and space for novelty, it is necessary.

Formlessness could be thought of as an inevitable phase where all that is known needs to be discarded to allow something new to be transformed with the contribution of the environment into having a potential of great richness. A reservoir that contains chaos, death, and destruction as well as the promise of a new form, full of liveliness, vitality and productivity. A phase of formlessness which includes creating while destroying, destroying while creating, comprised of chaos and ambiguity, is also sine qua non for creativity (Kaes, 2013).

Jan Abram (2013, p. 44) writes that formlessness had been added to Winnicott's vocabulary in his final years, although he had been exploring this

DOI: 10.4324/9781003380283-10

aspect of early psychic development from the start of his work. She also adds that formlessness is equivalent to his earlier concept of unintegration. Perhaps we can say that such a spontaneous, unintegrated way of being might not be limited to infancy but is a continuous, life-long possibility of psychic and mental functioning, of finding one's own being provided that there are significant others, and/or an analyst allowing such a psychic space of relating. Only out of formlessness and unintegration can a new integrated form, a true self, emerge (Abram, 2013, p. 45).

During infancy, the environment mother of quiet times who allows unintegration is integrated with the object mother who tries to meet the urgent needs of the infant with her reverie. Thanks to this, infants can be spontaneous and be themselves. In contrast, when infants, rather than the environment, have to adapt and there is a lack of good enough mothering, infants lose this opportunity to be spontaneous and be themselves. Instead, they have to erect defences to protect their core self such as false self, depersonalization, schizoid functioning, autistic defences etc. (Winnicott, 1945, 1960). Similarly, during adolescence, a good enough parenting/environment that can allow and accompany the natural formlessness of the adolescent is needed. An environment that doesn't try to give a form too quickly and prematurely to this formlessness and does not pressure for adaptability, is crucial.

According to Winnicott, searching for self can only come from natural nonpurposive, formless functioning in an intermediate area between the inner reality of the individual and the shared reality of the world where someone exists to have taken and reflected the communication of unintegrated self (Winnicott, 1971, pp 71–86). This points to a transitional space neither inside nor outside but in the space in-between, in relation to the other. Finding oneself can be realised within a good enough relationship.

Jacque Press (2013) points out that formlessness cannot be transformed unless there is a frame that contains it. Thus for this transformation to take place there needs to be parents who do not retaliate, who do not abdicate their roles and continue surviving in spite of the adolescent's aggression and destruction. The capacity to explore/find oneself and selfhood can only be achieved by an intrapsychically surviving object (Abram, 2022).

Formlessness cannot be transformed without a frame that contains it – a symbolic cradle. Jacquet & Huerra (2012) underlies the similarity of adolescent and infant needs with the "symbolic cradle" metaphor. Intense emotions are valid for both; parts of the body and psyche which are felt to be in pieces need integration and containing. Just as a cradle forms the boundary, protecting and holding the body of the baby from falling, or the arms of the parents which hold the baby emotionally and physically when in distress and crying, prevent the baby from disintegrating from anxiety, adolescents also need such a symbolic cradle. On one hand, boundaries, rules that will contain the adolescent physically in a private space (a concrete frame), on the other hand, an abstract nonphysical frame providing psychic containing, will form this symbolic cradle. Ogden (2009) emphasizes that in order for a person to be able to think his most disturbing thoughts two minds are needed, of course, this could also be two different parts of one's personality. All disturbing sensory experiences (betas) can assume a form, a shape and be transformed in this relationship. Only then will the adolescent be able to follow their passions and goals, and form an autonomous identity without early pseudo-maturation/individuation. A rigid pressurizing frame as well as too much understanding, and lack of boundaries will prevent adolescents from being themselves (Jeanmet, 2012; Kancyper, 2009). Only by displaying exaggerated behaviours, might adolescents protect themselves from merging with their parents and losing their identity. But it is not easy for parents to find this balance. Especially when they are usually going through their own midlife crises.

Working with adolescents

Working with adolescents requires one to be flexible, and able to tolerate uncertainty and sudden abandonment. The therapeutic process can be dramatic, vague and rapid. Especially at a time when adolescents are trying to be autonomous and independent, conforming to a psychoanalytic working frame might seem just the opposite of what they need. Coming to see an adult when they are trying to distance themselves from the adult world might also be challenging.

As Meltzer (1973) has stated that adolescents oscillate between different thinking modes and functioning worlds; an adult world that they might want to enter, a child's world that they want to leave behind, an adolescent world with their peers and also a space by themselves in isolation where they try to monitor themselves. An adolescent has not yet anchored in a single port, this is why an adolescent talking like a responsible adult one minute, might speak and act like an irresponsible child, needing protection, the next. A 14-year-old who attempts suicide, running away from home in the evenings, sending pictures of her naked self to boys and worrying her parents all the time by not answering her phone, at the same time, declares that her favourite thing to do is eat cookies while drinking milk and sleeping in her mother's arms. She also adds that she is afraid of sleeping alone. Adolescents themselves are tired, puzzled by these different, oscillating needs and affects, and feel fragile. Ernest Jones (1948, p. 387), says that "at puberty, a regression takes place in the direction of infancy and that the person lives over again though on another plane the development he passed through in the first five years of his life ... the individual recapitulates and expands in the second decennium of life the development he passed through during the first five years of life ...". Thus it is also a new chance to work through and transform remaining old conflicts from early childhood. But as Luis Kancyper (2009, p. 97) underlies "what is hushed up during childhood generally cries out during adolescence" so it is a phase where one will need to pay unpaid debts with interest. Harris's metaphor of "an internal war" going on where the enemy is inside, close and known seems very relevant (Harris, 1969). We listen to adolescents' changing discourses, their nostalgia for childhood, their struggle to take their first steps into adulthood, their anxieties, fears and possible obstacles in achieving this. We hear their conflicts as if listening to a polyphonic chorus, with all the psychic, bodily reactions evoked in us and all the associations that come up in our minds, images that come before our eyes (Anastasopoulos & Tsiantis, 1996). Anne Horne (2006, p. 154) uses the term "escapologists" as when working with adolescents we are usually not sure how much time we have before they might just run away/take flight. Adolescents want and at the same time do not want to come to therapy, they experience the conflict between dependence and independence. "Thinking" can also be perceived as something both persecutory and containing. A 17-year-old saying: "I do not want to think, what good is it any way to see, meaningless! I want to forget, not think at all but therapy makes me remember." This adolescent's resistance to see and think about his problems took a concrete appearance when he forgot to wear his glasses to his session making it nearly impossible for him to see the tip of his nose in actuality! Analysts can feel similar where oscillations such as coming closer or distancing themselves to the point of wanting to get rid of the adolescent as a result of feeling helpless and ineffective can occur (Segal, 1993).

The therapist, like the parents, might feel as if he is being tested by the adolescent, for his survival skills. When working with adolescents, one has to survive devaluation and abandonment without retaliation and continue going on being a solid container. One needs to keep in mind that destruction and aggression are healthy, normal aspects of growing up. What Winnicott said about the adolescent position as regards the parents could easily be applied to an analyst working with adolescents: "If the fantasy of early growth, there is contained death then at adolescence there is contained murder … growing up means taking the parent's place" (1971, pp 195). Analysts, similar to parents, need to manage without abandoning their roles, relinquishing principles or forcing adolescents to become adults prematurely. They also need to survive the adolescent's need to symbolically kill and achieve growth through the dead body of an adult.

What about the parents of adolescents?

Similar to when working with children, though it might depend and vary on the age and needs of the adolescent, one has to work with parents and take their transferences into consideration too. Unlike working with only the internalized parental figures of the adult, the parents of the adolescent are there in body and flesh, active in the adolescent's life and the therapeutic process. Though parents might not be seen as frequently as when working with children, it is not possible, nor functional to leave them outside the treatment as in adult work. Freud (1958) points out that there are few more challenges in life than trying to support an adolescent in becoming autonomous, and parents need help themselves. So while providing adolescents with an individual psychic space to help them form an independent identity, an authentic self where they can feel autonomous, the parents also need to be accompanied and supported in their role in assisting the adolescent on this journey (Novick & Novick, 2000, 2002a, 2002b, 2002c, 2013).

Akin to how adolescents are trying to find the right distance between themselves and their parents, in our work we also need to find the proper distance between adolescents and their parents. How often one sees the parents needs to be evaluated depending on each case's unique aspects/ dynamics and thus requires a certain degree of flexibility. Sometimes parents might want to manipulate the therapist just as they try to do with their adolescent, or might feel rivalry with the therapist when their feelings of insufficiency or inadequacy surface. They might idealize or denigrate, and test the limits of the therapist. In this regard, a great deal of attention needs to be given to transference-countertransference dynamics, including the parents, not only the adolescent.

Furthermore, in parallel to how the adolescent tries to find a place somewhere between the adult world and the child's world, an analyst working with adolescents might sometimes feel identified with the adolescent, that is to say, have negative feelings towards the parents, blame and criticize them or identify with the parents or become protective or punitive of the adolescent. All these feelings might affect the frame and result in leaving the parents out of the treatment or involving them too much, in short, not finding the much-needed proper distance (Godfrind, 1996). But we know that the way to meet these challenges cannot be reduced to simple ready-made solutions and that there cannot be one simple correct answer to deal with these complex dynamics. Working with adolescents we are aware that in our daily practice, very often we come across experiences where the situation is usually more complicated than what is obvious.

Concluding vignettes

I would like to give a case example of some of the fears, conflicts, and anxieties that might be experienced during work with an adolescent. My intention is not to present the case in all its richness and detail, but to simply introduce it in order to give body and flesh to the themes already addressed.

Hazel was a 16-year-old girl in 10th grade when she first came to see me. In our initial meeting to which she had come with her mother, she said that she didn't want her mum to come in and speak to me. She told me that although she has been feeling lonely, not wanted and unworthy since she was a child, things got worse particularly recently when she started high school and that's why she went to a psychiatrist and was given an antidepressant. Although she was a very intelligent girl, she was to fail her class which meant she would have to repeat or move to a state school in order to not lose the year. Later, she actually told me that even when she was just 4–5 years old, she had thought of jumping down from the balcony, but changed her mind as it wasn't high enough and she didn't want to risk being crippled.

Since her early childhood, she had been taken to psychologists for hyperactivity and attention deficit disorder and was recommended medication even then. But she never took medication nor received regular support. She thought she was an active, lively child, whereas her parents thought something was wrong with her. She was fed up of being compared to her much-adored older sister and complained of having grown up with babysitters, as well as very ambitious and hard-to-satisfy parents. She had to be number one in class and they always wanted more and more from her which made her feel as if whatever she did, would never be good enough.

She was the middle child and she had a younger brother for whom the mother gave up work at birth. He was, according to Hazel, the special one. She didn't actually have a room of her own for a very long time. It sounded as if she didn't exist, couldn't find her place in the family; between the older sister who was presented as the ideal one and the younger brother who was the special one. It was as if physical and psychic space for her were lacking.

It was striking to notice how her eyes kept looking, observing the room, every single object. Her eyes when directed towards the outside were perhaps a sign showing her wish to escape from exploring her inner world. We both thought that although it was in a negative way, her parents being called to school all the time might also be a way to be seen, to be noticed. Apart from her observant eyes, another thing that was noticeable since the initial meeting were the "gifts" she left in the consulting room; pieces of skin torn from her fingers, hair she pulled from her head, pieces of tissue, or an empty water bottle and one time, a bug. At first, she used to throw these items on the floor but later, rather than throwing them on the floor (even if she did that, she picked them up and piled them together afterwards) she started to make a ball of hair, sometimes also wrapped them around with a tissue, ball of tissue and left them on my table. Was this a way to show she existed, flesh and bone, a way to express her unconscious need to be contained with all her dirty, aggressive, violent and ferocious feelings, and fantasies? Her need to leave a mark on the other, even when she was gone? Similar to her self-harming, was it a way to prove and try to feel that her body was alive through pain, as she couldn't yet experience it as a source of pleasure?

On our second meeting, she came in with a tattoo on her arm which she was trying to hide from her parents by wearing a long-sleeved shirt. She said that two months ago she tried cold spray, cut her ankle and her wrist, that's when the counsellor at school called the mother to let her know of the situation. For our third meeting, she came in complaining about the "curfew" at home which was implemented as a result of her going out without her parents knowing, getting drunk, passing out, and having to be picked up by her mum. Meanwhile, her mum was saying that Hazel was going to kill her with all her disruptive behaviour; that she had a heart problem, and she couldn't bear this kind of behaviour. She kept telling Hazel that she could only heal if she got better. I felt that there was constant pressure from the mother; calling, mailing, wanting to cancel her daughter's session and come in her place. She was looking at me with expectant eyes after each session and was also saying that she just couldn't physically and emotionally/psychically bear it. In fact, she fainted after one of her daughter's sessions and had to lie down for quite a while in my office to recover. This young girl had difficulty controlling her aggressive impulses, thinking about her deep anxieties and psychic pain she instead wanted to escape and evacuate all those mentally and emotionally unprocessed feelings by acting out. But it seemed that her environment was far from providing a containing frame too. Mother was overwhelmed with panic and father was almost absent. I had hoped that the psychiatrist I had referred the parents for consultation would see and support them regularly but when this failed, I referred them to another colleague with whom I could be in contact and work in cooperation, and who could see the parents, acknowledge their needs, support them in their parenting in a regular frame. Meanwhile, the psychiatrist was handling the medication of the adolescent. The parents didn't continue with the colleague for parent work but continued meeting with the counsellor at school and the psychiatrist. During the process, we also had meetings with both parents and the adolescent present, some mother-daughter and some father-daughter sessions.

At the beginning of our work, while she was speaking, I can vividly remember how an image of a *jelly-like figure*, very slippery and difficult to hold, formed before my eyes. Could this image be a production of her unconscious projection/transference of how formless she feels herself to be, of not having a particular shape and, how uncontained she might be feeling in object relations? I think it was after seven or eight sessions, I had a dream: "taxi dream". In the dream we are having the session outside the consulting room, near a shopping centre quite near to where I live, talking on the way. We stop a taxi together, and just when the two of us are going to get in, she makes me get in first, and then closes the door and signals the taxi to leave and then she gets into another cab. I feel panic, where did she go, how will I find her, what will I tell her parents? I think this dream reflects many aspects of how I feel working with her; wanting to work and perhaps not wanting her at the same time, wanting to get rid of her because of all the anxieties she evokes in me and finding it hard to deal with her acting outs pressure from the parents, the overall difficulty in containing it all and mobilizing infantile defences against helplessness. How long will she stay with me, will she just be like she is shopping at a store, coming in trying out some outfits and then leaving? Could it reflect the anxiety regarding uncertainty and an unclear working frame, vague boundaries? These feelings are also what this young girl needs to evoke in those who are close to her, her parents, counsellor, psychiatrist and of course, her analyst. Perhaps it could also be important that the analyst initially has these dreams and feels panic in her place, for this young girl is in deep pain, whose inner world is full of violence, disappointment and hopelessness. In fact, after a short while, Hazel started bringing dreams representing the fragmentation, disintegration, violence and panic in her inner world.

There were periods where just before our first separation she told me that she had swallowed ten pills the previous night but nothing happened, another incident where she had to be hospitalised due to an alcohol coma, a psychotic breakdown where hallucinations and delusions appeared, leaving a suicidal note at school, right after she didn't get the attention she wanted from the school counsellor. Of course, though addressed to the counsellor, the note referred to her anger, and frustration, perhaps to everyone; her analyst, parents, all the adults who couldn't seem to protect her, who are useless. It was also a call for help, a desperate need to be seen and recognized.

It felt as if we were in some sort of a "survival programme", being tested for skills of endurance. During the process, acting-out continued in various ways but decreased in frequency and intensity. To feel helpless, alone, and unprotected was so painful that separation and loss needed to be denied immediately, evacuated by action so as not to think about it or turned into verbal attacks about my incompetence during our session. It was striking how any kind of emotional pain couldn't be tolerated, thought about, but instead acted out. She couldn't mourn for the lost object, but rather devalued it, and turned it into rubbish. I was very often seen, especially after breaks, as a useless, worthless person who met with her only for the money. Similarly, all the feelings she projected into me were exactly how she felt herself to be. She thought of herself as rubbish, disgusting, destructive, and bad and this is perhaps why she always wanted to leave marks (dirty marks) in my room. She touched, and mingled everything in the room; for example, her hands all over my table leaving fingerprints everywhere; she squeezed paper in between the table, her drink about to spill all over the place. Her way of making people remember her, was not by loving, caring, affectionate bonds, but her destructiveness, devaluation, her badness. As if saying "I am a disgusting person and you will remember me with my disgusting marks, and bad doings. One thing she wouldn't tolerate would be to be forgotten, to be just among the bunch of ordinary adolescents. So at school, she also did everything to be noticed, like sleeping in class, not handing in homework, not attending class, or exams, to be visible to the teachers, creating and wanting a privileged status. While I was trying to contain all these feelings sometimes I felt insecure, helpless and not being able to think. But this blockage in me was also a way to understand the difficulty Hazel experienced in thinking about herself. She seemed to express herself as if only moments existed, nothing before or after, bits and pieces. Not much of a connection which would lead to integration, narration. We talked about how important it is to be able to connect things, past-present, experiences. Importance of trying to give meaning, to have a story, which would lead to integration. Otherwise, there were moments, holes, just scenes, without connections. In line with this, whenever I was interested in what she was telling me or wanted to make a link she always said in an irritated, sarcastic way, "What's the importance of it, why is it important?" and cut me off. As if she needed to attack all kinds of linking. I thought that it was if she were trying to prevent me from forming a thought in my mind similar to her own experience perhaps of not having a combined, functional and containing couple. It was as if she were trying to prove that no one could put up with her and saying, "Let's see how much longer you would be able to tolerate me." Was I going to be like the mother who fell ill and was fragile, who collapsed whenever Hazel expressed anger? Or like the father who denied his feelings and distanced himself? There were times that I found myself close to both positions. Right after those sessions where I thought we had come closer and allowed a space for thinking, there were usually acting outs and an attack, as if even starting to feel hopeful was dangerous and must be killed off immediately. I myself had to experience what she was feeling, contain those feelings and survive. The more I could contain these destructive feelings within me without retaliation, the more she felt secure and trusted that I could symbolically hold and contain her. Being able to notice and think about the feelings such as the anger, hatred and hopelessness that this young girl evoked in me, helped me to be able to integrate them with those of love, compassion and protectiveness.

She started telling me: "I always hated doing whatever I was told as if it would mean losing my independence. I don't want to be good or proper, so I do something to ruin that and then I am relaxed. But recently, I am a bit distanced from doing whatever comes to my mind. Although I still think about cutting myself, I stop it and control myself, wait. Actually, when these thoughts come to my mind I can write now. I also prefer to read, can listen to music or watch series to pass those moments."

A dream content with a different tone follows, very different compared to earlier dreams which were full of raw material, and of disintegration: "I was on my bike trying to ride on a very narrow path where there are thorns. I keep falling and hurting myself, my knees etc., bleeding. I am trying to head towards the school, there are houses of tissues. I go to these houses to care for my wounds. There are also mountains between the path and the school, so I leave my bicycle but I climb over the mountains and reach the school."

Actually, I thought about this dream, as quite positive, and different in tone, compared to other dreams she had been telling me, where there were usually men following her, trapping her in a tunnel, tying her up, cutting her legs, and arms, opening up her abdomen etc. We talked about the parallelism of what she told me about school being her best option. She is riding the bicycle, and in spite of the falls, wounds, and bruises, she is not giving up. She reaches a place with structure.

Eventually, there came a time when she started emptying her handbag and showing me all that was inside or showing photographs that she had taken, her new hobby. She began to share her inner world where she had the courage to explore her psychic life, her gaze directed inside than outside.

Fortunately, as her therapy progressed, she started to verbalise her frustration regarding separations, and when in a session I told her about the cancellation of her two sessions in the coming month, she was able to tell me how she fantasized about killing me. So gradually, it became possible for her to verbalize her frustration, and anger at being left rather than her turning it against herself and acting out.

When working with this young adolescent, I felt as if we were on a rollercoaster; rapid ascending, descending, suddenly stopping and going in reverse, a back-and-forth journey. On the one hand wanting to feel the rush and bear it but at the same time, wanting to get off as soon as possible. This resembles the two different functionings, two different voices in her. One part wants to forget, deny everything and denigrate any help offered to her, just wants to quit. Another part recognizes her needs, wants help and demands change. A psychotic part relying on omnipotence, and a neurotic depressive part which feels pain. As our work progressed the latter became more audible. A new character emerged in the sessions; a tiny kitten that she started to look after: a baby creature who doesn't let her sleep and wants constant attention and gets her claws out and scratches immediately when not being attended to. But also a resilient little kitten who does not give up trying to come up to her bed although she throws her out. Just like her. She arrives at one of our sessions looking devastated, nauseous, saying that she had to lie down on the couch. She feels relaxed on the couch, and although at first, I have no idea what has happened to her, eventually I understand that her kitten had become ill which made her feel very guilty. She tells me that she feels incapable in everything and that she couldn't even look after her kitten. She adds that it's like she damages everything she touches. She asks me why she has to struggle so much all the time, not to harm or do something stupid to herself. It is striking that she couldn't express her sorrow or her tender feelings regarding her kitten face to face but rather on the couch, where she wouldn't need to see me. We talk about her behaviour of going to a bar and drinking so as not to feel pain, as a way to silence, and freeze her sorrow about her kitten. I am also deeply moved and find myself hoping that the kitten survives.

After this session, I had a dream about my patient. In my dream, Hazel is brushing her teeth and then empties her mouth on me. Then she lies down on the couch, and I tell her that I can contain in my mind all her vomit, shit and all her fantasies about killing me, but won't allow her to kill me in reality! As it could be understood from the dream, the path is full of thorns and to contain all that is projected is not that easy. All the unprocessed feelings that weren't worked through come up in the dream. One can easily see we are more than just a mirror onto which patients project their internal figures and to whom we react. We need to be open to all kinds of feelings and allow our minds to be affected too. But also we need to have a thinking and understanding space to contain and have a distance from these feelings. To "use our countertransference as a servant and not as a master" as Hanna

Segal (1981, p. 20) points out meaning that while we are deeply involved and affected, at the same time we need to be uninvolved and detached, using countertransference as a guide to understanding what is going on in the patient and in the interaction between us, rather than acting under its influence. Working through the strong emotions projected into us, being aware of and processing our countertransference, and not being lost in all the feelings that are evoked in us, is a way to keep ourselves and our patients alive.

This adolescent girl, her kitten and the analyst managed to survive ... In order to psychoanalytically survive, means to preserve the capacity to continue thinking, it becomes crucial to think together with colleagues, and intervision, supervision is so significant. Hatred of the patient, omnipotence, withdrawal, which can all be triggered by our infantile defences as a reaction to our feelings of helplessness, can be thought about but not acted upon. Also, not being alone in these cases when acting out of the patient is frequent, cooperation with the school, psychiatrist and family is important and necessary in therapeutic work. In an analytical process, in order to enable our analysands to have the courage to look inside themselves, we also need to be alert to the images that appear before our eyes, to phantasies, and dreams, and to our physical reactions while continuing to look deep inside ourselves. Forming intimacy in any relationship, including a psychoanalytic one, and within oneself requires that, as analysts, we remain unafraid to look deeply at our countertransference experiences. Only then can we help others to have an intimate relationship with themselves so that a transformation can take place.

References

Abram, J. (2013). On Winnicott's area of formlessness: The pure Female element and the capacity to feel real. *European Psychoanalysis Federation Bulletin* 67: 43–57.

Abram, J. (2022). *The Surviving Object: Psychoanalytic Clinical Essays on Psychic Survival-of-the-Object*. London: Routledge.

Anastasopoulos, D. & Tsiantis, J. (2003[1996]). Countertransference issues in psychoanalytic psychotherapy with children and adolescents: a brief review. In: *Countertransference in Psychoanalytic Psychotherapy with Children and Adolescents*. EFPP Clinical Monograph Series. London: Routledge, pp. 1–35.

Freud, A. (1958). Adolescence. *The Psychoanalytic Study of the Child* 13(1): 255–278.

Freud, S. (1937). Analysis Terminable and Interminable. *International Journal of Psychoanalysis* 18: 373–405.

Godfrind, J. (1996). The Influence of the Presence of Parents on the Countertransference of the Child Psychotherapist. In: *Countertransference in Psychoanalytic Psychotherapy with Children and Adolescents*. EFPP Clinical Monograph Series. London: Routledge.

Harris, M. (1969). On Learning to Know Oneself. In: *Adolescence*. London: Karnac Books, p. 3.

Horne, A. (2006). Brief Communications from the Edge: Psychotherapy with Challenging Adolescents. In: Lanyado, M. & Horne, A. (eds), *A Question of Technique:*

Independent Psychoanalytic Approaches with Children and Adolescents. London: Routledge, pp. 149–165.

Jacquet, Y. & Huerra, P. (2012). Conversions. In: A.G. Kuëy (ed.), M. Işıl Ertüzün and P. Jeanmet (trans.) *Adolescence: Landmarks for Parents and Experts*. Istanbul: Bağlam p. 35 (published in Turkish).

Jones, E. (1948). Some Problems of Adolescence. In: *Papers on Psycho-Analysis*. London: Maresfield.

Kaes, R. (2013). Formlessness, The Group, Training. *European Psychoanalysis Federation Bulletin* 67: 173–182.

Kancyper, L. (2009). Adolescence as a Dynamic Field. In: Ferro, A. & Basile, R. (eds), *The Analytic Field*. London: Karnac Books.

Meltzer, D. (1973). Adolescent Psychoanalytical Theory. In: *Adolescence*. London: Karnac Books, pp. 22–29.

Novick, J. & Novick, K.K. (2000). Parent work in analysis – children, adolescents, and adults: part one: the evaluation phase. *Journal of Infant, Child & Adolescent Psychotherapy* 1: 55–77.

Novick, K.K. & Novick, J. (2002a). Parent work in analysis II – children, adolescents, and adults: recommendation, beginning, and middle phases of treatment. *Journal of Infant, Child & Adolescent Psychotherapy* 2: 1–27.

Novick, J. & Novick, K.K. (2002b). Parent work in analysis – children, adolescents, and adults. part three: middle and pretermination phases. *Journal of Infant, Child & Adolescent Psychotherapy* 2: 17–41.

Novick, K.K. & Novick, J. (2002c). Parent work in analysis – children, adolescents, and adults: part four: termination and post-termination phases. *Journal of Infant, Child & Adolescent Psychotherapy* 2: 43–55.

Novick, K.K. & Novick, J. (2013). Concurrent work with parents of adolescent patients. *Psychoanalytic Study of the Child* 67: 103–136.

Ogden, T. (2009) *Rediscovering Psychoanalysis: Thinking and Dreaming, Learning and Forgetting*. London and New York: Routledge.

Press, J. (2013). Formlessness, the intimate, the unknown. *European Psychoanalysis Federation Bulletin* 67: 28–37.

Segal, H. (1981). Countertransference. In: *Counter-Transference, Theory, Technique, Teaching*. London: Karnac Books, pp. 13–20.

Winnicott, D. (1945). Primitive emotional development. *International Journal of Psychoanalysis* 26: 137–143.

Winnicott, D. (1960). Ego Distortion in Terms of True and False Self. In: *The Maturational Process and the Facilitating Environment*. Madison, CT: International Universities Press.

Winnicott, D.W. (1971). *Playing and Reality*. London: Routledge.

11 Social withdrawal in adolescence

Psychodynamic reflections and clinical strategies

Thomas Marcacci

Introduction: social withdrawal in adolescence: the importance of extending both the object of analysis and the analytic subject

In this chapter we will reflect on an insidious and serious manifestation of psychological distress that manifests critically in adolescence: social withdrawal.

This phenomenon refers to complex situations, where multiple factors are at play that can be observed from multidisciplinary perspectives: psychodynamic, psychiatric, and sociological (Berman & Rizzo, 2019). Here, necessarily, we will focus only on one perspective of observation, that is, deep psychic dynamics, dwelling on some of the factors at play, deferring considerations from different perspectives to other occasions. Scientific advancement, indeed, is the result of partial contributions, in a team effort.

There are two main concepts I would like to put forward for consideration here. The first is how social withdrawal can be understood as a particular manifestation of adolescent breakdown. The other, how it is a situation where the horizon of the psychic to analyze must be extended in space and time. With respect to this, in my view, even the analytic subject must likewise extend. I mean, on the one hand, that the object of treatment may not only be the patient as an individual but also the relational environment where he lives. On the other, that in order to do this the individual analyst will not suffice, nor will mere extemporaneous collaboration between professionals, by juxtaposition, let us say. There is a need for a further level, namely the consolidation of the equipe as a working group, so that it constitutes itself as a true analytic subject. We will deepen these concepts in the course of the chapter.

Theoretical frame

Forms of withdrawal meant as difficulties in object investment, in all their degrees of severity, and relationship-related difficulties are as early as object encounter is, and are, therefore, present well before adolescence (Jacobson, 1964). It is at this developmental stage, however, that they can take on additional criticality, tying in with some of the most important developmental

DOI: 10.4324/9781003380283-11

tasks of this phase of life (Blos, 1962): separation from the family unit of childhood; acquisition of an individual identity by finding a place in the peer generation; integration into the Self of the developed body and of genital sexuality. The obstacle to these dynamics, at a life stage that is not just a moment in time but an organizing agent of the mind (Cahn, 1986), charged by the renewed drive intensity that puberty brings, makes the manifestations of social withdrawal in adolescence a particularly critical symptom. In the conviction that any analytic reflection can only be rooted in clinical experience, some case examples will accompany us on our journey.

Social withdrawal in adolescence, as we have noted, is a varied phenomenon that can occur along a gradient of severity. We can imagine at one extreme the situation of a young boy who magnifies his stomach ache just a little to stay home from school, remaining for a day in the reassuringly comfortable warmth of his room. This is a situation in which we do not see a criticality at all and with respect to which, indeed, we might even empathize, with a hint of nostalgia. Proceeding in an aggravating sense along this gradient of symptomatic manifestations, we can imagine, for example, situations in which the ache begins to become no longer consciously magnified but actually perceived, albeit without any organic basis, associated with an anxious state of varying intensity, without the possibility of a thought that gives it meaning. In this situation, the teenager may begin to miss more days of school and perhaps even retreat from other social settings, sports or other activities, due to perceived or anticipated anxiety of experiencing out-of-control feelings of malaise. Here, progressing toward severity, the child may begin to build a defensive barrier to protect himself from contact with the environment, distancing himself from it physically and psychically. He begins to envelop himself in self-isolation, where he can feel and discharge excitement without the complication and the fear of meaningful objectual bonds, especially with peers. Or, in a different way but to the same end, where to defuse such arousal a priori, withdrawing from the risk of it being solicited by the relational context.

It is like wrapping oneself in a cocoon. This, from a certain point of view, can be considered a useful defence if used as protection at a time when the transformation of identity through puberty and adolescence upsets and makes one feel vulnerable and if, therefore, the subject perceives that he needs time to allow personal evolution to mature, following its own internal rhythm, which may be different from that required by the environment. In this case, we can imagine this cocoon as permeable, a membrane that doses and allows contact with reality, rather than interrupting it. In more problematic situations, however, this cocoon of isolation may be an airtight capsule, which protects the subject but at the price of stifling his developmental possibilities, removing the exchange with the environment that is the necessary nourishment for all evolution (Winnicott, 1965).

It is the latter situations, in particular, that provide a breeding ground where a psychic functioning of the schizotypal spectrum can easily come to the fore and develop. Some of these situations, then, may extend and consolidate towards, frankly, psychotic functioning, perhaps remaining for years below a pathological threshold as positive symptoms but festering as negative symptoms and structuring a psychotic potentiality, to use the words of Aulagnier (1975). There are several recent and large-scale epidemiological researches, such as the one conducted by the European research group EU-GEI (2014), that indicate how these pathological potentials of the schizotypal spectrum functioning develop, or fail to develop, toward an established psychotic functioning and structure because of concurrences in complementary series between genetic, environmental, as well as between intra- and transpsychic dynamics.

I propose here to consider the psychic situation of severe social withdrawal as one of the manifestations of breakdown in adolescence: there is withdrawal from reality rather than breaking contact with it, as in a psychotic crisis; self-disuse and deactivation of the intensities at play rather than irrepressible expression of them and fragmentation of the self; suspension of time rather than derailment from the path. We could call it abeyance instead of breakdown. Opposite phenomenologies but with the same meaning: breakdown of the evolutionary relationship between subject and environment.

Social withdrawal, or abeyance, as I propose to call it here, is a particularly insidious psychic situation because it is made up mainly of negative symptoms that remain elusive. It is an extreme defence aimed at protecting one's sense of self not by psychotic change of reality but by distancing oneself from it through suspension of time and space. These are situations that proceed silently, where awareness of the severity is slow to be recognized. Therapeutic alliances very slow to form, precarious and often interrupted therapeutic contacts, lack of patient and parental compliance. Cleavages and denegations of the patient and his primary relational environment are projected into the context, whether social, institutional or clinical, fragmenting it and hindering its ability to think and hold.

Over time, the teenager's self, deprived of the nourishment and developmental stimulus provided by contact with external reality, becomes a karst, fragile ground, ready to collapse in the face of a stress for a reality that easily becomes excessive. This situation of withdrawal can remain crystallized for many years, as in the fairy tale of "Sleeping Beauty", or lead, under a reality stress that shatters the defence of withdrawal, to decompensation, when by then psychosis has taken root.

In its various forms, what we are discussing in this chapter is a widespread and growing symptomatic situation, at least in post-modern Western societies (Lyotard, 1979). In some countries, such as Japan, it has long been a phenomenon studied from multiple perspectives (Kato , Kanba & Teo, 2019). In others, such as Italy, my home country, the horizon of the problem is only just beginning to be defined. In early 2023, for example, the first survey by the Italian National Research Council (IFC-CNR, 2023) came out, providing a quantitative estimate of the phenomenon, which was found to affect, in its severe form, 2.6 percent of 15- to 19-year-olds. Males are actually more withdrawn but more females perceive themselves as such. The phenomenon, however, is difficult to quantify, remaining by its nature largely undeclared and inconspicuous until its most critical manifestation. For example, one parent out of four accepts the serious withdrawal of the teenager without reporting it or making it problematic.

This phenomenon, on the one hand, has general psychic dynamics underlying it, regardless of the patient's country of origin, on the other, there are important cultural differences. This is precisely because of the importance, for understanding this symptom, not only of intrapsychic or family dynamics but also of the resonance between these and psychic elements deeply sedimented through generations, specific to any given culture. Therefore, a dialogue between colleagues from different backgrounds will be particularly valuable here.

While social withdrawal in adolescence is not yet a specific syndrome included within the DSM-5 (APA, 2022), there may be many criteria for establishing a threshold of criticality, regardless of the presence of positive psychotic symptoms. For example, Kato, Kanba & Teo (2019), with respect to the Japanese context, propose as an inclusion criterion for Hikikomori syndrome a withdrawal to one's home lasting for six months.

In this chapter we will consider as a critical threshold a continuous and established withdrawal from school attendance. This, in fact, still represents an important dividing line of severity, negatively impacting several developmental tasks proper to adolescence, as we saw earlier, and acting as a flywheel for further problems. Furthermore, the interruption of school attendance is likely, in these cases, the moment that makes explicit the malaise that, often, until that point has remained repressed or denied.

Let's begin by observing some clinical situations, on the basis of which to make some reflections.

Gina is an 11-year-old girl enrolled in the sixth grade. Her parents have been separated for several years but are still entangled in jealousies and grudges that hinder their ability to cooperate in their relationship with their daughter. Gina began struggling to go to school as early as the end of fifth grade, the year she began pubertal development and had her first period. She complained of somatic symptoms with respect to which any organic cause was ruled out. This year, starting from the first months of school, she has attended rarely, building up to complete discontinuation. She has similarly withdrawn from dance classes and refuses opportunities to meet with friends. Somatic symptoms are no longer present but for her firm opposition, with respect to which her parents are in check.

She agrees, however, to come to therapy, although for a long time it will only be possible to see her once a week, due to both her and her parents' resistance. In the sessions, however, her presence is massively shielded behind a false self: she shows me an idealized image of herself, projected mostly on her own past experiences. She brings me the outfits she used to dress up in as a princess at carnival when she was younger and photographs of when she was participated in the end-of-term ballets. She tells me in detail how various choreographies should be done, or how she could cook perfectly, or how easy it would be for her to achieve good results at school. But actually she does none of these things. This crude reality is unthinkable for her and she splits off the part of herself that is felt as inadequate and shameful, and projects it outward, onto her peers. "Chiara [former dance partner] is negated for dance, she just can't do it, she misses even the simplest steps. She is pathetic." One can hear the ruthless, dismissive coldness in her voice when she tells me this. An atmosphere of tension and judgment descends in the session that I feel pressing down on me, as if I cannot miss a step as well. I myself feel blocked by this judgement, like a cat in front of a dog, which is ready to attack it at the first sign of weakness.

We can hypothesize that this internal voice, acted out by Gina against parts of herself projected onto her friend, emanates from an intransigent Super Ego, which attacks and humiliates the sense of self experienced by Gina herself, judging it to be inexorably lacking in relation to an Ideal Ego out of reach. As a defensive reaction, she has structured a False Self (Winnicott, 1965), idealized and divorced from reality, behind which she screens herself. Experiencing aspects of the Self other than idealized, well-functioning, smiling ones is not sustainable for her. We might speculate that the gap between ideal and real does not cause her a little tolerable frustration that would be growth-promoting but, rather, a depressive meltdown that is too frightening. External contexts or stimuli that tend to bring Gina into contact with her real limits provoke a strong anxiety reaction and are drastically rejected, as they are perceived as a threat to the defensive balance with which she wants to protect herself. Reality, and in particular the authentic mirroring that can be received in peer contexts, must be kept at a distance.

We can draw from this first example to advance some general reflections.

The first concerns the salience of an aspect that I have found in every clinical situation of social withdrawal that I have treated: the patients' experience of such a huge gap between an ideal expectation and a fragile sense of self that it is deemed unbridgeable; this unbridgeable gap inhibits contact with reality. The expectation with respect to this contact, indeed, is a narcissistic wound that puts the whole Self at risk of collapse. With respect to this risk, even a real, and therefore by definition not ideal, satisfying experience is not a sufficient counterpart.

We can advance the hypothesis that this is precisely a central point with respect to both understanding and treating these clinical situations, as we shall see later.

It is important to reflect, in each specific case, on what is the role of different psychic instances with respect to the patient's experience of self-inadequacy. What is the relative weight of the Super Ego in bringing to the Self a particularly crushing experience, demanding an Ideal Ego in a sadistic and humiliating way. How heavy is, instead, the individual narcissistic fragility, sedimented through the intrapsychic layers of personal evolution, with respect to which the patient's Ego Ideal does not stand as a useful spur, regardless of the quality of superegoic pressures. Or what, rather, is the role of a Super Ego Ideal, transpsychic content emanating from others' expectations, near or far in time or space, intrusive and alienating for the patient's Self and acting from within. The consideration of what relative weight these instances have on the psychic horizon with which we are dealing will be crucial in guiding our intervention.

A further critical aspect in these clinical situations is the patient's relationship with his own body, as highlighted by Laufer & Laufer (1984) in their now-classic work on adolescence and developmental breakdown and as explored by numerous subsequent works, including, for example, those of Italian authors such as Nicolò and Ruggiero (2016).

Greta is frustrated for the loss of familiarity acquired with the body of childhood; she realizes that, through puberty, the idealized self-image she had previously, of a light and agile dancer, finds opposition from the reality of a body that escapes control, for it takes on dimensions and characteristics different from those desired. Withdrawal from the context of peers also becomes, for her, a rejection of the mirroring they can do for her changing body.

"I looked in the mirror and I saw myself crooked. I really feel that my neck is not growing straight. I try to straighten it, twisting it like this. Sometimes I hear a 'click', I feel straighter, but then, instead, I see myself crooked again. I can't go out and be seen crooked." These are the words of Anton, a 16-year-old patient, whom we will meet better in a moment, and they express very clearly the experience of an inadequate evolution of the Self. An experience which is not thought but felt in the body, of being incorrect, unpresentable and of being despised if his backbone is not straight. We see the precariousness of the sense of self, swinging from the illusion of security to shame in the blink of an eye.

Subjective disconnection from the passage of time seems, indeed, to be another aspect that recurs in similar situations. Time seems suspended, with the unconscious fantasy of controlling the development of the body and the evolution of social identity, like putting a movie on pause. In particular, the future seems disconnected from the self: there are at best isolated desires, like floating rocks in the middle of a void, with no thinkable path to arrival.

Clinical intervention

Let us continue by beginning to consider possible strategies of clinical intervention with respect to these situations.

A first element that stands in the way of treating these patients is the difficulty of establishing and maintaining therapeutic alliances. Since the psychic functioning hinges precisely on withdrawal as a defence, it is evident that this will also affect the relationship with the analyst.

A key variable with respect to the therapeutic course will be, therefore, whether the patient is able to have direct contact with the analyst. This crucially affects the form that the therapeutic course may initially take. Furthermore, it is an indicator of the balance between the intensity of patient's defence and his resources to evolve.

I stand with other authors (Erlich, 2019) in considering that therapeutic contact doesn't regard only the patient's ability to physically go to the analyst's consulting room but that it could also take advantage of long-distance communication tools that can offer initial avenues of engagement for these situations, a sort of transitional space, with opportunities and limitations (Lin, 2015). Furthermore, the construction of therapeutic contact should also include the possibility of the analyst himself moving toward the patient.

Another example will aid us here: At the beginning of our journey, Anton's bond with me and with the therapy was weak. The contact between us extended and deepened very gradually and in a nonlinear way. Over time, we have managed to build the possibility of seeing each other for three sessions a week but skips and periods of interruption are always present.

We have now reached the second summer break and Anton is struggling to return to therapy. This happened after previous breaks as well, with him saying: "Well, I don't know, I'm just busy these days. Actually, I don't think I need therapy anymore; I've been fine on my own." This time, however, the situation seems different. At the resumption, he doesn't come and doesn't respond to those messages that I've sent to him over several weeks.

Based on previous experience, I had suggested that he schedule a couple of phone sessions through the summer break, but he missed those appointments. He flunked last year, with the narcissistic wound to him and his family that this entailed. I know that he had not had much social interaction with peers during the summer. After a couple of weeks of silence I decide to call his parents. They say their son had experienced no critical moments over the summer and the psychotic symptoms he had some time ago have not reappeared. However, he is increasingly withdrawn, and saw his friends only rarely over the summer. He is now locked in his room all day playing computer games. Together with his parents, I consider visiting him at home. I keep in mind the risk that he might experience it as an intrusion into his protected place and I would myself feel much more comfortable in the safe zone of my consulting room. I decide to go anyway, alerting him both by text and through his parents.

On the first occasion he keeps his bedroom door shut. I speak to him from the outside: "Hello Anton. We haven't seen each other for a long time and I am very curious to get your updates. If you'd like I'm here." I stood waiting outside his door, adding afterwards: "When we see each other frequently and then for a long time there is absence, we could be disoriented, like something is missing; one could be a little bit angry too. Does it happen to you as well?"

He doesn't open nor speaks. Next time, however, he opens the door and allows me to watch him play on the computer, showing me how the character in his role-playing game has evolved.

After these two "home" meetings, Anton was able to resume the sessions.

With other patients, of course, such an out-of-setting approach would constitute an inappropriate action. I believe, however, that this therapist's move toward the patient could be necessary in these situations. Don't get me wrong, I am convinced that interpretations of the most acute anxieties taking place in the here and now of the session are crucial and are the most transformative tool even in the analysis of severe adolescents. However, in the very particular developmental situation of a withdrawn adolescent, I believe that in some delicate stages of bond building, making the patient feel a surplus of object investment towards him by the analyst can help the former to invest in the therapy. Feeling sought for and considered by the analyst, for his wellbeing and vital parts, can, in my opinion, help to limit the patient's fear of his own vulnerable and blocked parts. Furthermore, this could make him feel less scared of dependence on the other which, especially in adolescence, is as much feared as sought. The analyst is invested by the patient's projections of powerlessness. Moving outside his comfort zone and going toward the patient could be seen as an enactment, an interpretative action (Boccara, Materangelis & Riefolo, 2018): an experience which the patient could share, perhaps identifying with the possibility of not giving up but seeking a way out precisely through contact with the other.

An important reflection could be opened here on how the psychic dynamics that drive social withdrawal are linked to the digital experience in adolescence. Such reflection deserves a dedicated space that cannot be delved into here. We must limit ourselves to noting how the personal and social experience that teens have in the digital realm can either be a useful transitional space, if used as a protective filter but with a view to evolution, or instead entail risks of entanglement, creating an addiction that hinders growth. Withdrawal into the digital is more likely to be the defensive consequence than the cause of severe social withdrawal; although, then, like any addiction dynamic, it can take on pathological significance in its own.

This example makes it clear how the setting is intensely stressed in these situations. We move, here, into a borderland of our discipline with respect to both theoretical considerations and clinical techniques. As analysts we are here at a crossroads: either we intercept only those patients who are already able to fit the classical setting that we have envisioned, or we explore further horizons for the analytic practice (Cooper, 2005; Green, 2012; Bastianini & Ferruta, 2018), seeking tools to expand its theoretical and technical frontiers and boundaries and, with them, our range of patient interception. As analysts, our challenge will be, in this case, trying not to lose a proper analytic approach. It will be important, for example, even in these situations "off the couch", to build a setting, both as an invariant that allows us to grasp the dynamics of transference-countertransference, and as an elaborative container for the projections of the patient's split parts (Bleger, 1967; Collovà, 2013). I anticipate here the proposal that this setting could consist of the clinical equipe, as we will see better later.

In treating these clinical situations, the parents of withdrawn teens are very frequently the initial link and, for a long time, may remain the only avenue of intervention in this situation.

It may be that the need for a psychological consultation arises directly from them, or it may be prompted by some institution, usually the school, that has picked up the teenager's and the family's malaise. These three eventualities, whether the teen succeeds in coming to the analyst, or not and the parents bring the problem themselves, or, finally, whether it is an institution outside the family that raises the problem by urging therapeutic contact, will already give an important indication of the seriousness and resources of the situation.

Initial consultations with parents will provide valuable information for guiding the subsequent work. In addition to trying to get a sense of how serious the adolescent's situation is, with respect to symptoms, functioning, and psychic structures, it will be important to discuss with the parents if their child is able to put himself on the line, sufficient enough to give the therapeutic bond a chance to form. Otherwise it will be worth continuing to see the parents.

From Anton's example above, we could glimpse the usefulness or, actually, the necessity of involving parents in treatment, not only from a legal and practical point of view but precisely from a clinical perspective as objects of the analytic intervention. They are subjects involved in a blocked relational field (Ferro & Basile, 2007). It is necessary, therefore, to consider what valence the dynamics within the family bond may have and whether transpsychic elements may play a significant role with respect to the individual's situation. Several authors have highlighted from different theoretical perspectives such dynamics: Pichon Rivière (1980) with the concept of "vinculo", Racamier (1990) with that of "enmeshment," Kaës (2015) with that of "bonding".

In these clinical situations, as in any serious psychopathological situation, the dynamics underlying it lead on one hand to a striking symptomatic manifestation in one of the family members but, on the other, extend beyond it, in space and time, both with respect to etiopathogenesis and consequences (Faimberg, 2005).

Victor is a 19-year-old boy whom I have been treating for two years, now with the frequency of three times a week. Only at this stage of therapy has he become able to look back on his past, retracing the years when his crisis began. He says: "In middle school I was good at soccer, I remember being nice to my friends, being a bit of a child and they saw me as a good boy. Then I moved on to high school and it's like I lost myself. I didn't want to look naive by being good, I didn't come across as likable anymore. It was like my body didn't respond to me anymore either: before I used to play soccer naturally, then it was like I had to think about every movement as if it was new. It has been a very difficult year, I remember feeling terribly lonely, as if I didn't even have the company of myself. My parents didn't understand it at all, they were just asking me about school, about grades. But I resisted, I managed to stay at school, and toward the end of the year I had begun to find a new way of being with my classmates. I was satisfied with me for that and I thought that if I was overcoming these difficult things it meant that I was growing up. That's when my parents told me that in order not to risk flunking out, they were going to sign me up to an easier school. It was the same school where I had gone to kindergarten when I was little. At that point, everything fell apart for me. I don't know what happened, I was starting to feel older when suddenly I felt small again."

This example can make us reflect on two critical issues. The first is the friction function that parents perform between their child and external reality. In the course of the son evolution, from birth to full adult autonomy, it will be necessary for this parental function of friction to evolve, calibrating to the child's growing possibilities of taking charge of a direct contact with reality and, at the same time, pushing him in that direction. Taking our cue from the above example, we can observe how the parents' conscious desire for protection, if not calibrated by an empathic closeness with the child's experience, does not function for him as a defence against the shocks of reality but rather risks precluding him from authentic contact with it. This contact, indeed, in sufficiently tolerable forms, is indispensable for obtaining an authentic sense of self through the experience of having been tested.

The other central point that needs to be considered, as we saw earlier with respect to the consideration of the relative role played by Super Ego, individual narcissistic fragility, and Super Ego Ideal, is which unconscious pressures and expectations are conveyed beneath this parental function. In our example, we can reflect whether underneath the explicit desire for protection acted out by the parents, may lie the unconscious desire, on the part of one or both of them, to conform the child's life to their own expectations, projected onto him. These expectations could involve the son continuing to remain dependent on them or conforming to their ideal, for their own narcissistic gratification. The child's narcissism rests on what is lacking in the realization of the parents' dreams of desire, as Kaës (1993) reminds us.

With respect to this, that the child can take ownership of his own history, giving it a meaning that enables him to become aware of his personal developmental path, is a key moment with respect to self-identification and differentiation from the parents' perspectives and meanings.

Let us now examine the parents' perspective, using another clinical example.

When Alex's parents come to me, concerned about their 23-year-old son, the situation they tell me appears immediately to be very serious, with frankly psychotic symptoms that seem well-established. After listening and trying to understand Alex's present situation, I try to ask the parents about the path that led him to this point. They tell me that when he was in the fourth grade, aged 17, out of the blue, he ran away from school one day, seized by an anxiety attack. Since then he has not returned to school and before much longer he retreated to his room. Now he hardly leaves home. I tell them, "It's been six years, what has happened in this time?" Here, I suddenly encounter a chasm of emptiness. They look at me wide-eyed, as if they have only now realized how much time has passed. Says the father, "Six years … but how was it possible that so much time has passed. What have we been doing all these years?" He asks turning to his ex-wife, "I don't know … I try to think about it but now it's as if my mind has gone dark, I have no memory of us in those years," she says.

I have now been following them weekly for several years and have been able to see the emotional, relational, cognitive resources they both have. Yet, at the beginning of our journey those six years were a black hole, lived and unexamined (Bollas, 1987), so dense that thought had not yet been able to experience it. In our path, slowly, together we have been able to contact the distressing experiences of those years: their separation; the collapse of the hope of having, as a couple and as parents, a reparative experience with respect to relational bereavements with their families of origin; the ghost of living again, as parents, the contact with mental suffering, after having experienced it in their past as children or as siblings, a ghost too frightening to be thought about, acknowledged, treated at the time it was forming.

I think this example can show well how transpsychic dynamics in such important relationships as family ones can intertwine with the intrapsychic dynamics of the individual patient. This, of course, applies universally; however, while in other situations we can afford to circumscribe the scope of analysis to our relationship with the patient in the consulting room, dealing only with the psychic derivatives that appear in the session, in complex situations such as social withdrawal in adolescence it becomes imperative, in my opinion, to bring the environment around the patient into the horizon of analysis. By environment, I mean first of all the parents but also the adolescent's main social contexts.

Together with other authors, such as Mastella & Ruggiero (1999), I find it necessary that, in situations like Alex's, there should be one therapy for the adolescent and one for the parental couple, which should go in parallel, with two different analysts.

The hypothesis behind this belief is, as we have seen above, that the psychic dynamic underlying social withdrawal is strongly intertwined with certain developmental tasks specific to adolescence: individuation, separation from childhood parents, subjectification and peer socialization of developed body and genital sexuality. Actually, these dynamics are not only developmental tasks for the adolescent but equally prompt an evolution in the parents, as individuals and as a couple. They, too, will be urged by their child's changes to face an identity transition. The transition from a relationship with a child, hinged on primary caregiving and on the dependence this creates, to one with an adolescent, made up of growing autonomy, differentiation, ceding control. This creates new spaces also for the parents. This, just as for the adolescent, can also cause parents to experience a mixture of relief and bewilderment, longing and mourning. The drive storm that accompanies puberty and adolescence can expose parents themselves to question their own sexuality, couple satisfaction, and change in their ageing bodies.

In mental situations as severe as social withdrawal in adolescence, we cannot run the risk of not taking charge of the other fundamental subjects of the primary bonds in which the teen is embedded on a daily basis. The possibility that the subjective situation is, certainly not only but also, the catalyst for projections from the environment, in the present or across generations, must be considered and, if need be, managed. Otherwise, when, as Racamier (1986) says, in family ties the interactional register prevails to the detriment of the intrapsychic one, an evolutionary possibility that may germinate in one of the actors in the field will remain in check against the difficulty of the others to evolve likewise.

It should also be noted that is frequently the case in these situations that parents are separated. We know that separation may also interfere with the developmental and subjective process of the adolescent child (Cahn, 1998). If parents fail to keep their bond firm with respect to the parental function, despite their division as a couple, the separation may become a critical element. This is both with respect to the mourning of the whole family for the dream of a solid and satisfying union, and with respect to the greater difficulty separated parents may have in sustaining each other's role and in integrating their different perspectives on the child. The blind spots in this disunited triangle and the collusions that arise from time to time between the teen and one of the parents to the exclusion of the other, may become a fertile ground where the child's withdrawal consolidates. An analysis could help to regain or to consolidate the parental functioning, even if not as a couple; at the same time it will help both parents to evolve with respect to the stresses placed on their role at this delicate stage.

We should now move toward another very important consideration. Always, but particularly in developmental age, we must keep in mind the importance not only of the patient's internal world but also of his external environment and of the objective time of his life. Some developmental transitions, indeed, can and should be caught in a given space and time, outside of which some doors risk closure by the objective harshness of reality.

This leads me to emphasize how important it is, in these clinical situations, that one of the clinicians of the equipe takes care of the connection between the family and the environment outside it. On the one hand, it will be essential to keep in touch with the institutions involved, especially the school. On the other, it will be necessary to consider and coordinate the opportunities of experience and socialization that the environment can offer to the teen, if necessary with the accompaniment of an educator. In the equipe, indeed, the presence of this latter professional figure is, in my opinion, as necessary as the others, in order to accompany the patient when he resumes moving toward the otherness, at the same time protecting and stimulating him.

This brings us to one of the pillars of clinical intervention in these situations: offering the withdrawn adolescent a constant, challenging and sustainable pull toward sociality. The most important element of this action that we could call "traction toward the world" is, in my opinion, its dose. This must be calibrated subjectively, day by day, and this becomes possible only on the basis of a sufficient knowledge of the internal dynamics of the subject involved and of his relational environment; sufficient knowledge which could be matured within the analytic path and deepened through the team discussion. It is an essential part of the clinical strategy that the interventions of all clinicians are coordinated by a constant reflection within the team itself and not only proposed following the perspective of each individual profession.

The equipe's effort to reach this closeness and attunement with the patient will offer the teenage an experience of narcissistic reinforcement that will provide him with valuable fuel to resume evolving. I repeat here as well, how I consider this only part of the necessary work, the other part being constituted by the elaboration, in analysis, of the deep-seated anxieties that can sabotage this possibility of feeding on good experiences, and by the elaboration of the non-developmental bonds in which the family is stuck (Bion, 1962). We cannot dwell on this here, however, I would like to emphasize how for these situations one of these interventions without the others is incomplete and risks remaining sterile: provision of the narcissistic reinforcement that comes from mirroring an authentic element of the Self that the subject can recognize and on which he could base his move forward; transformation of the deep-seated anxieties, intra- or trans-psychic, that hinder the integration and evolution of the Self.

In the equipe so far we have seen different roles: analyst of the adolescent, analyst of the parents, community therapist who, for example, could be the same analyst as the parents' one, professional educator. Another clinician who must, without doubt, have to be part of the team is, of course, a psychiatrist. Although the situations described here show mainly a massive presence of negative symptoms, which are less treatable pharmacologically, while the positive ones remain subthreshold for a long time, nonetheless the latter can occur and phases of more psychotic decompensation can enter the horizon. The possibility of a discussion between analyst and pharmacologist with respect to the understanding and management of the symptoms is fundamental. Similar symptoms, even with severe manifestations, may have different psychic causes and purposes. Aspects of communication, compensation of compromise, and biochemical mechanism are interwoven together. Reflecting together on the relative weight of these aspects allows a better grasp of whether and when to intervene pharmacologically or, in cases of necessity, even with hospitalization, or whether it is possible rather to understand and contain the symptoms within analysis and teamwork.

Finally, there is the subject of the treating team, in my opinion the most important of all in these complex clinical situations: the equipe itself. This is precisely what I mean here, when I refer to the need to extend the analytic subject. The equipe can constitute itself as a third subject, composed of individuals but exceeding their mere sum. This is provided that the team takes care to constitute itself as a working group, committing itself in the long run to building a habit of shared thinking and management of clinical situations, through intervisions at constant and continuous frequency. In a team used to working together, it creates a mutual knowledge of each other's psychic functioning. Trust fosters with respect to the group's constructive elaboration of members' contributions. Even further, on this basis, inter-psychic (Bolognini, 2019) and bodily (De Toffoli, 2016) resonances are created which allow the team to grasp deep levels of contact with the psychic environment it is dealing with. Over time, across the cases treated, constant elements sediment within the team and become known. These constants go on to constitute a setting, meant as an invariant with respect to which grasping the dynamics elicited by the encounter with the patient and his environment. Here, strengthened by this setting offered by the team, the individual analyst can afford to explore a little beyond the boundaries of what would be his individual setting.

A group that is not used to working together but meets extemporaneously to discuss a clinical case will likely struggle to constitute itself as a setting and will have fewer tools to catch and prevent acting out and splits.

The equipe constitutes itself as a second-level container, with respect to the individual analyst; a container that integrates and signifies the experience that each individual team member has with the patient. Moreover, the team, as a subject in itself, receives and sometimes enacts precisely the most split, most distressing and most non-integrated parts of the patient. Parts that exceed each individual's ability to grasp and contain them. This is not only because of an excess of quantity over the psychic possibilities of an individual, but because of the essence of these projections, which concern not only intrapsychic contents but relational patterns, functioning of the bond and spaces in the background to it. We can think, therefore, that the equipe can supply a more effective containment experience, precisely because it is a metapsychic subject (Kaës, 2009), constituted by the structure and functioning of the bond between its members, and because the understanding, containment and transformation of the evolutionary possibilities of the analytic field occurs also through the very functioning of the team bond.

Dealing with situations of social withdrawal, there are various dynamics with respect to which the team can constitute itself as a transformative container of distressing experiences, split off and projected into the context by the various individuals involved.

The environment around the teenager is, usually, permeated by a sense of loneliness, powerlessness, frustration, emanating directly from the patient's experience. The projection of this experience brings the risk of fragmenting the environment, for it is received along with the very defensive mechanism to keep that experience away. This pushes the actors involved to a schizo-paranoid functioning. The equipe is not exempt from the same pressure. Having consolidated the team functioning over time will help to capture and contain these dynamics. The individual therapist will himself feel fully powerless and experience narcissistic frustration in the face of these cases. However, he will be helped to bear these experiences and to regain a realistic sense of efficacy by seeing his own contribution, though partial and limited, becoming more effective because of the joint action of all. This experience of teamwork that enhances everyone's specific contribution, will be an important antidote to the sense of deep loneliness that easily permeates the actors in these contexts.

To conclude: many things remain to be said about these complex clinical situations which are impossible to elaborate on here. We have highlighted some aspects of the intrapsychic dynamics of the withdrawn adolescent. We have highlighted the imbalance between his sense of self and his ideal expectations, reflecting on the different roles that Super Ego's characteristics, subject's narcissistic quality and Super Ego Ideal could play for this imbalance. We have observed the teen's difficulty in integrating the developed body and in fitting into the flow of time.

In respect to the intervention, we proposed the importance of team work and of attuning each intervention on the evolutionary possibilities of the field. In doing so, we highlighted the importance of building an equipe, not only as a second layer container for the single clinician, but as a setting and, furthermore, as a metapsychic subject.

References

American Psychiatric Association (APA) (2022). *Diagnostic and Statistical Manual of Mental Disorders* (5th rev. edn). https://doi.org/10.1176/appi.books.9780890425787.

Aulagnier, P. (1975). *La violence de l'interprétation: du pictogramme à l'énoncé.* Paris: Presses Universitaires de France.

Bastianini, T. & Ferruta, A. (2018). *La cura psicoanalitica contemporanea. Estensione della pratica clinica.* Rome: Giovanni Fioriti Editore.

Berman, N. & Rizzo, F. (2019). Unlocking Hikikomori: An interdisciplinary approach. *Journal of Youth Studies* 22(6): 791–806.

Bion, W.F. (1962). *Learning from Experience.* London: William Heinemann.

Bleger, J. (1967). Psycho-analysis of the psycho-analytic frame. *International Journal of Psycho-analysis,* 48: 511–519.

Blos, P. (1962). *On Adolescence: A Psychoanalytic Interpretation.* Glencoe, IL: Free Press.

Boccara, P., Meterangelis, G., & Riefolo, G. (2018). *Enactment. Parola e azione in psicoanalisi.* Milan: Franco Angeli.

Bollas, C. (1987). *The Shadow of the Object.* New York: Columbia University Press.

Bolognini, S. (2019). *Flussi vitali tra Sè e Non-Sè.* Milan: Raffaello Cortina Editore.

Cahn, R. (1986). *Psychoanalyse adolescence et psychose.* Paris: Payot.

Cahn, R. (1998). *L'adolescent dans la psychanalyse.* Paris: Presses Universitaires de France.

Collovà, M. (2013). Il setting come luogo delle trasformazioni possibili. In: Ferro, A. (ed.) *Psicoanalisi Oggi.* Rome: Carocci Editore.

Cerrai, S., Biagoni, S., & Molinaro, S. (2023). Hikikomori: indagine sul ritiro sociale volontario dei giovani italiani. Istituto di Fisiologica Clinica del Consiglio Nazionale delle Ricerche (CNR-IFC), Gruppo Abele, Università della Strada, Pisa. https://www.gruppoabele.org/documenti/schede/report_hikikomori_rev_aggiornamento16_01.pdf

Cooper, A.M. (2005). *The Quiet Revolution in American Psychoanalysis: Selected Papers of Arnold M. Cooper*. New York: Brunner-Routledge.

De Toffoli, C. (2016). *Transiti corpo-mente*. Milan: Franco Angeli.

Erlich, L.T. (2019). Teleanalysis: Slippery Slope or Rich Opportunity? *Journal of the American Psychoanalytical Association* 67(2): 249–279.

European Network of National Networks Studying Gene-Environment Interactions in Schizophrenia (EU-GEI) (2014). Identifying Gene-Environment Interactions in Schizophrenia: Contemporary Challenges for Integrated, Large-scale Investigations. *Schizophrenia Bulletin* 40(4): 729–736.

Faimberg, H. (2005). *The Telescoping of Generations: Listening to the Narcissistic Links Between Generations*. London: Routledge.

Ferro, A. & Basile, R. (2007). *The Analytic Field: A Clinical Concept*. London: Karnac Books.

Green, A. (2012). *La clinique psychanalytique contemporaine*. Paris: Ithaque.

Istituto di Fisiologia Clinica del Consiglio Nazionale delle Ricerche di Pisa (IFC-CNR) (2023). *Hikikomori: indagine sul ritiro sociale volontario dei giovani italiani*. Online edition, available at www.gruppoabele.org/documenti/schede/

Jacobson, E. (1964). *The Self and the Object World*. New York: International Universities Press.

Kaës, R. (1993). *Le group et la sujet du groupe*. Paris: Dunod.

Kaës, R. (2009). *Les alliances inconscientes*. Paris: Dunod.

Kaës, R. (2015). *L'extension de la psychanalyse*. Paris: Dunod.

Kato, T.A., Kanba, S. & Teo, A.R. (2019). Hikikomori: Multidimensional Understanding, Assessment, and Future International Perspectives. *Psychiatry and Clinical Neurosciences* 73(8): 427–440.

Laufer, M. & Laufer, E. (1984). *Adolescence and Developmental Breakdown. A Psychoanalytic View*. New Haven: Yale University Press.

Lin, T. (2015). Teleanalysis: Problems, Limitations, and Opportunities. In: Scharff, J.S. (ed.), *Psychoanalysis and Psychotherapy in China*. Psychoanalysis Online2. London: Routledge.

Lyotard, J.F. (1979). *La Condition postmoderne: rapport sur le savoir*. Paris: Éditions de Minuit.

Mastella, M. &Ruggiero, I. (1999). L'intervento "combinato" con adolescenti e genitori nelle crisi adolescenziali. *Interazioni* 13(1): 34–54.

Nicolò, A. & Ruggiero, I. (2016). *La mente adolescente e il corpo ripudiato*. Milan: Franco Angeli.

Pichon Rivière, E. (1980). *Teoria del vinculo*. Buenos Aires: Nueva Vision.

Racamier, P.C. (1986). L'intrapsychique, l'interactif et le changement à l'adolescence dans la psychose. In Baranes, J.J. & Cahn, R. et al. (eds), *Psychanalise, adolescence et psychose*. Paris: Payot.

Racamier, P.C. (1990). A propos de l'engrénement. *Gruppo* 6: 83–95.

Winnicott, D. (1965). *The Maturational Process and the Facilitating Environment. Studies in the Theory of Emotional Development*. London: The Hogarth Press and the Institute of Psycho-Analysis.

Index